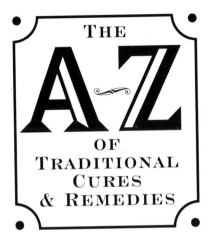

THE
A-Z
OF
TRADITIONAL
CURES
& REMEDIES

THE

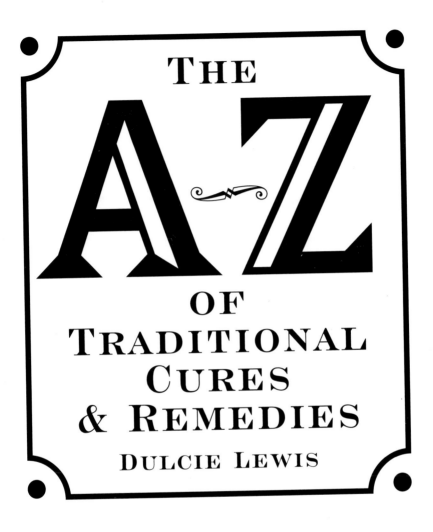

A-Z

OF
TRADITIONAL
CURES
& REMEDIES

DULCIE LEWIS

COUNTRYSIDE BOOKS
NEWBURY BERKSHIRE

First published 2002
© Dulcie Lewis 2002

Reprinted 2003

COUNTRYSIDE BOOKS
3 Catherine Road
Newbury, Berkshire

To view our complete range of books,
please visit us at
www.countrysidebooks.co.uk

ISBN 1 85306 766 0

Cover design by Nautilus Design (UK) Ltd
Line illustrations by Trevor Yorke

Produced through MRM Associates Ltd., Reading
Printed by Borcombe Printers plc, Romsey

INTRODUCTION

Maxims of Health – 1848
Keep the head cool
The feet warm
Take a light supper
Rise early

The huge popularity of Family History groups and the research undertaken in tracing our ancestors reveals much about our relationship with the past. We are now in an age where families are smaller and often isolated, without the support network of aunts,

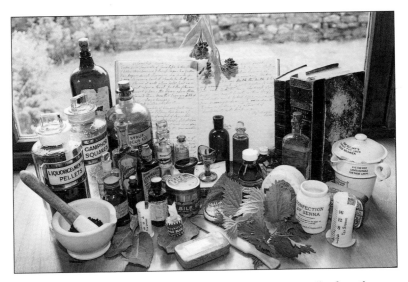

A collection of old medicine bottles, ingredients and patent remedies from the recent past. All the old favourites are here: senna, liquorice, camphor, syrup of figs, camphorated oil and chlorodyne. Bottles containing poison were usually green and had vertical ridges as a warning for the blind or those who could not read. Blue bottles were preferred for syrups. (Photograph Ann Holubecki)

uncles and cousins, where we are unlikely to know the person living across the road; somehow faced with this we are trying to establish a link with those who went before us.

A family likeness from an old sepia photograph, an ability or weakness, a health problem; all may recur through the generations linking us to a bigger whole than our immediate nuclear family. The more we delve into our own history, the more we value the efforts of those in the past who worked to keep a roof over their head, food on the table, their children properly clothed and with at least an elementary education. However, for me and for you too perhaps, otherwise you would not have picked up this book, it goes further. My middle name is Margaret and my female cousins too share this name. My paternal grandmother insisted that each of her daughters-in-law should keep the name in the family. Margaret was the name of her only daughter among six sons, who died aged 11 during a meningitis epidemic in the early 1900s. Many of you will have such reasons for your names.

I admire and am intrigued how people in the past struggled to keep their families well and in as good health as possible, given their lack of our modern day drugs and medical procedures. These are not far distant generations for there are many today who recall being treated when ill with items from the kitchen cupboard and common wayside herbs.

A lady who told me of some Suffolk remedies recalled: 'As children it was a treat to be ill. When we had a bad cough or cold a fire was lit in our bedroom and lavender burnt on the fire to get rid of smells. Mother rolled brown sugar into balls and a mixture of honey and vinegar was sipped a little at a time. If we had difficulty swallowing she boiled onions in milk and mixed them in with lots of bread and plenty of pepper. I still like bread and milk when I'm not well.'

Before the introduction of the National Health Service in 1948, with free medical help for all, any treatment by a doctor cost money. Therefore most families attempted some healing for themselves. Cures that appeared to work were passed round by word of mouth and noted in commonplace books. I have tried to record here the ingenuity of our forebears in using and adapting for healing what was around them. One stands amazed at the intuitive pre-penicillin use of such things as cow dung and mouldy bread!

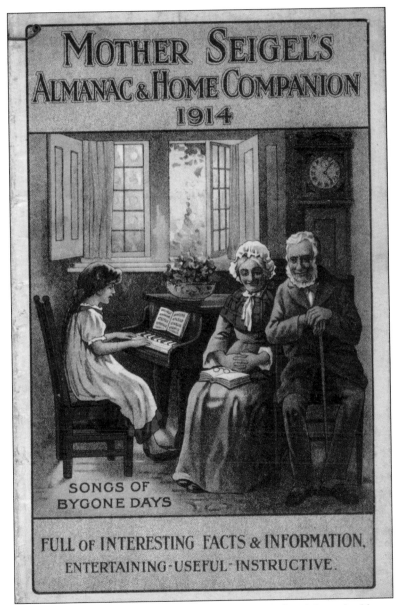

Ordinary people relied on these little home remedy books for advice on health, medicines, baking and home hints. Often they were given away free to promote a patent medicine, in this case the Mother Seigel range. Others were produced by salesmen who sold them from door to door. (By kind permission of the Thackray Museum, Leeds)

Among ill-educated people in remote country areas, more in touch with nature and the seasons than those living in the towns, there was a strong belief in superstitious healing rituals and charms. Isolated areas where the next village was many miles away, as in parts of Devon, Cornwall, Yorkshire, Northumberland and Shropshire, were the most susceptible to health superstitions. Many were an odd combination of Christian symbols and old witchcraft – hedging their bets you might think. They were often supplied with cures by the local 'wise woman' or a travelling pedlar or quack doctor. I have attempted to record some of these old superstitious 'cures', but toads and teeth found in churchyards are of only limited interest in this cynical age. I could have filled a book with wart cures alone!

There was no shortage of medical advice in the past; from Culpepper's *The English Physitian* of 1652 through to John Wesley's *Primitive Physic* of 1747. Later there were large numbers of popular self improving Victorian journals, almanacs and pamphlets such as that written by Dr Henry Smith in the late 1800s, W*oman; her Duties, Relations and Position.*

For the first half of the 20th century medical advice was available from the little home remedy books, price around 1/-, sold from door to door and ordinary people relied heavily on these publications. They have proved a rich source for many of the cures in this book and I am very grateful to the people who gave me old family copies found when they were clearing out a loved one's belongings.

Patent medicines made fortunes for those who were clever enough to market and sell what was in most cases a laxative, and many made extravagant claims as regards healing. The home remedy books promised to save you money by providing a list of the ingredients for well known patent medicines so you could visit the local chemist and have them made up at half the price. In earlier times you might have paid an apothecary for some herbs or a tincture for you to make your own nostrum.

Doctors openly advertised their books, pamphlets and pills in the newspapers. A Dr Vernon of Kentish Town said of his own essay, 'It may be justly considered the GREATEST MEDICAL WORK OF THE AGE'. His capital letters, not mine!

Many doctors were happy to give a long range diagnosis without ever seeing the patient. This advertisement appeared in the *Teesdale Mercury* in 1875 from a Dr Barnes of Lonsdale Square in London:

'Important to Country patients. He may be consulted personally or by letter for the benefit of nervous Sufferers who cannot visit him. He is ready to give his opinion upon the nature of the case and the principle of treatment necessary to effect a perfect cure.'

The rich were almost more disadvantaged than the poor for they could afford medical treatment – and oh how they were treated! Doctors could see pound, shilling and pence signs over every rich sick bed and gave 'heroic' doses of powerful medicines and procedures. The rich were spared nothing; bleeding, purging, leeches, vomits and enemas were all administered when all that might be needed was a light diet and some peace and quiet.

We learn something of this from the Mildmay account books. The Mildmays were a rich and influential family who, at one time, owned most of Chelmsford in Essex. In 200 years they rose from a stall in Chelmsford market in the 1500s to important positions at Court and marriage to a cousin of George I. Benjamin Mildmay, Earl Fitzwalter showed a keen eye for financial detail and recorded:

'December 21 1747 – Mr Truesdale, apothecary, his bill in full to Xmas 1745 – £86 2s 6d.
March 6 1748 – Gave Dr. Beaumont for attending me 5 or 6 times in order to remove a little complaint in one of my eyes – £4 4s – veritable charlatan.'

Members of the aristocracy and royalty were served the most harshly of all, for many were treated with cruel procedures as each doctor saw honours and riches within his grasp if his medicine succeeded in a cure. Royalty were often prevented from a dignified death by their doctor's administrations. It is the only time that the humble cottager with a few herbs was better off than the suffering rich.

I have therefore, in some instances, included the professional advice you might have received from a doctor to put in context the home remedies being tried. Many were infinitely preferable to the 'heroic' treatments being given to those who could pay for their medicine.

Some of the remedies will make you smile, others will appal you. I am loathe to refer to 'old wives tales', being an old wife myself, but there was a basic wisdom in many of the old cures and a self-reliance that is to be admired. A GP remarked to me once that his surgery was full of young mothers with small children lacking the basic knowledge or instinct of how to treat a slightly raised temperature.

Those readers born before 1950 will remember many of the medical myths I have recorded. Those born after that date will wonder how we could possibly have believed in them.

My collection of remedies is primarily from our recent past but in some cases it stretches back to our forebears' frantic efforts to keep clear of the Plague. This book is not an exhaustive list of every potion swallowed or ointment rubbed on. A bread poultice was the same whether made in a Tyneside terrace or a Cornish cottage. I have kept my reference to toads to a minimum.

Perhaps I should finish by saying what the book is not about. It is not another treatise on herbs and their uses and I have only written about the herbs I have come across in actual remedies. Neither is this a manual on homeopathic or alternative medicine; there are many experts and books on those branches of medicine to consult if you are interested. It goes without saying that I neither recommend nor have I tried any of these cures.

My sole aim is to open up and give a glimpse into that part of everyday life with which our ancestors coped daily – how to keep well. I have tried to give meaning to names, medicines and ingredients long fallen from use and to explain simply the illnesses that were feared and which to us now seem just so much part of history.

Dulcie Lewis

ACKNOWLEDGEMENTS

I have received so much generous help with this book that I am bound to leave out someone who should be mentioned. Short of visiting every county in England I had to ask friends – or friends of friends! – to research information for me in their particular county. Grateful thanks to all the following, and there is no need to dread another telephone call from me: Barbara Arm, Joy Calvert, Patricia Carpenter, Barbara Cox, Rita Craske, June Graham, Susan and Ian Hardaker, Ann Holubecki, Irene and Joseph Irving, Helen and Malcolm Loft, Lorna Martin and Pauline Stevens.

Others who did not know me but were generous in their help were: Kate Wills and The Living Memory Group of Northampton; Stan Hill, Editor of *The Blackcountryman* magazine; Jean Howard and David N. Robinson of the Louth Naturalists' Antiquarian and Literary Society, Lincolnshire.

Anyone interested in the history and development of medicine must pay a visit to the lively Thackray Museum, Beckett Street, Leeds. Alan Humphries, the Librarian, was very generous in sharing with me his encyclopaedic knowledge of this subject.

Thanks too must go to the following: Barbara Blakeson, Curator of Human History for the Harrogate Museums and Art Gallery Service; Rosemary E. Allan, Senior Keeper at Beamish Open Air Museum, Beamish, County Durham; Ruth McKew at the Salt Museum, Northwich, Cheshire; the ever patient librarians at my local library in Leyburn, North Yorkshire and also to the library services at Cheltenham, Leamington Spa, Malvern and Margate.

Finally, I would like to thank my husband Ray who dutifully kept 'the band in the nick' while I neglected all housewifely duties to write this book.

A

To eat an apple going to bed, makes the doctor beg his bread.

ABORTIFICANT. Certain herbs taken to excess were said to bring about an abortion. However, they were also likely to poison you. See **parsley, pennyroyal, rue** and **slippery elm**.

Drinking hot **gin** in a hot bath.

An excess of **purgatives** such as **aloes** and the patent medicine **Mother Seigel**'s Operating Pills were a common household method of abortion.

ABSCESS. A site of infection characterised by redness, heat, swelling and pain. Once pus has formed heat can be applied to the skin to bring the abscess to a 'head'. Men over 60 have painful memories and bear the scars still of a hot **poultice** made either of flour and hot treacle or **bread**, **soap** and sugar. Placed by a vigilant mother onto an abscess this agonising home treatment would successfully burst the abscess and release the pus. See also **groundsel**.

AGE. Without doubt we aged earlier in the past. Poor working and living conditions, chronic illnesses that failed to kill but reduced you to the state of a permanent invalid, all contributed to early ageing. The spry 70 year olds circling the globe on long haul holidays today would reject completely the following definition from a 1930s home recipes book, 'Old age in women sets in at 53, in men about the 60th year.'

AGRIMONY. *Agrimonia eupatoria*, also known as sticklewort or cocklebur. A common wayside herb with anti-inflammatory effects, and used since Anglo Saxon times for healing wounds. The flowers can be cut and dried and used in an **infusion**.

John Wesley's *Primitive Physic* recommended washing putrid **wounds** morning and evening with a warm **decoction** of agrimony and 'apply a **poultice** of the leaves pounded, changing them once a day 'till well'.

Agrimony was also thought to be good for regulating the function of the gall bladder and kidney and **liver** complaints.

An early 20th century home remedies book advised, 'The best comforter for a depressed or desponding mind is equal parts of **agrimony** and **rosemary**, made and used in the manner of tea.'

AGUE. An older name for **malaria** but often used to describe a shivering fit. Ague was in common use in Shakespeare's time and in *Twelfth Night* he named the pompous courtier Sir Andrew Aguecheek. Relief was to be had 'When the fits are on', by taking an egg in brandy and going to bed.

ALEXANDERS. *Smyrnium olusatrum* or black lovage. A recognised medicinal herb from the 16th to the 19th century. Looking not unlike celery and growing on cliffs and hedge banks in the South and Midlands, these plants were once found in every monastic garden. The seed soaked in wine promoted menstrual bleeding, though what the monks were doing concerning themselves with this remains to be seen.

The leaves were a remedy for **scurvy** and the roots are mildly diuretic. William Coles in his 16th century book *The Art of*

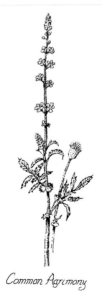

Common Agrimony

Simpling wrote, 'The leaves bruised and applied to any bleeding wound, stoppeth the blood and dryeth up the sore without any grief.'

ALCOHOLISM. In Victorian England cheap alcohol and public houses opening all day from early morning meant many people passed a miserable life in an alcoholic haze, neglecting and often abusing their families. The awful prospect of the workhouse loomed for the whole family when the breadwinner was no longer able to work. The Temperance movement encouraged people to give up alcohol and Nonconformists signed The Pledge but what to do if you were too far down the slippery slope?

J. T. Butterworth in his *Practical Medical and Commercial Recipes* of 1897 wrote: 'It is often a difficult problem to know what to do with a confirmed toper. To steady a man who has been drinking heavily, a wineglassful of **vinegar** or a full dose of liquid ammonia acetate is remarkably effective. Caffeine and Coca Wine have recently been advised to cure dipsomania. Rigid abstinence from alcohol and a stay in a home for a lengthened period of time affords the greatest hope of a cure.'

A simple country cure was drinking the water in which **horseradish** had been boiled.

ALOES. Also known as **bitter aloes**. A bitter purgative drug made from the dried leaves of various species of aloe found mainly in southern Africa. It acts mainly on the **bowels** and was often used with **soap**, or iron and strychnine in the treatment of **constipation**. See also **Mother Seigel** and **Whelpton's Vegetable Purifying Pills**.

AMBER. A form of pine oil derived from the fossil resin of extinct coniferous trees and considered by herbalists to be good for rubbing on the chest for **colds** and treating an upper respiratory tract infection.

ANAEMIA. The most common form of anaemia is due to a deficiency in iron. Women particularly suffer at times due to pregnancy or heavy periods.

The Lady's World of 1898 saw it as a problem of the servant class and this extract gives a dark picture of life below stairs. 'Domestic

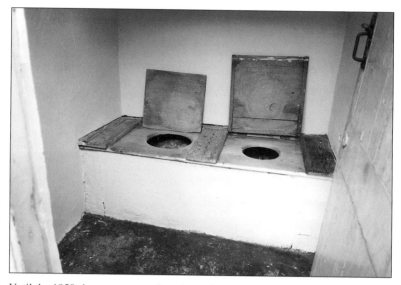

Until the 1950s huge amounts of aperients, laxatives and purgatives were taken on a regular weekly basis. Besides lack of roughage and not drinking enough water, could the outside privy have contributed to the country's constipation? A typical outdoor brick built 2 holer bucket privy, although this one is quite up market with the hinged lids.

servants have to work for many hours at a stretch and much of that work has to be done in the lower, darker rooms of the house. Their food is often of coarse quality and of insufficient quantity. Lastly their meals are usually hurried and taken at irregular intervals. Girls and young women employed as servants are particulary liable to suffer anaemia, indigestion and ulcers of the stomach.' No mention was made as to how this state of affairs might be overcome.

A simple country cure from Northamptonshire, unlikely to do any good, advised the anaemic girl to go out in the early morning and smell the sheep in the fields. However, country people also knew the tonic effect of **nettles**.

A homemade tonic for anaemic women: 1 quart of Tarragona (a port in north east Spain) wine, a jar of Bovril, extract of malt and 3 pennyworth of **quinine**. Scald the Bovril and malt with 1 pint of boiling water. When cold add the other ingredients and mix well.

A small glass every morning.

Small fortunes were to be made from the patent medicines containing iron and there were plenty from which to choose:

Warner's Safe Cure for Women
Widow Welch's Female Pills
Pink Pills for Pale People
Ayers **Sarsaparilla**
Strengthening Medicine for Delicate Girls
Blaud's Pills

ANAESTHETIC. Early civilisations knew the deadening effects of **opium**. In medieval times in England anyone attempting an amputation would have administered a 'knock out' brew of wine containing briony, hemlock, **henbane** and **opium**. Later this mixture was superseded by a liberal amount of alcohol.

The muscle relaxant nitrous oxide, or 'laughing gas' as it was known, was discovered in 1795 but its uses in surgery went unrecognised. Ether was not used as an anaesthetic in England until the middle of the 19th century and was followed very shortly afterwards by chloroform, often administered by a hospital porter holding a rag and a bottle of chloroform.

ANKLES. For curing weak ankles John Wesley's *Primitive Physic* instructed the sufferer to plunge them into cold water for 15 minutes morning and evening. The circulation may well have benefited from this rather abrupt treatment. However, by the 1900s the method was more refined when the advice was that twice a day the ankles should be sponged with salt water and then rubbed dry for 15 minutes.

ANTIMONY. A toxic metallic element commonly known as tartar emetic, because of its powerful purging properties. Antimonial wine was once used in the treatment of **bronchitis** as in very moderate amounts it eased a cough. However, in large amounts it produces vomiting, purging and in some cases even paralysis.

ANTIPHLOGISTINE. A popular treatment for **pleurisy** or congestion of the lungs right up to the Second World War. A grey compound, looking not unlike chewing gum, bought from a

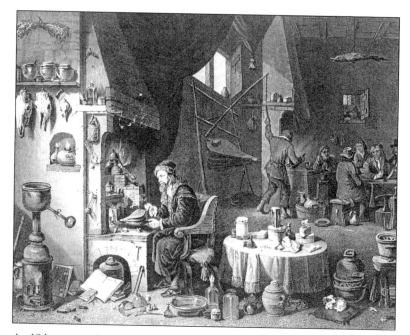

An 18th century view of an apothecary at work. He would supply native herbal medicines but also potions and ointments with more exotic ingredients brought from abroad. Sometimes an apothecary might also trade as a grocer or a chandler and dabble in a bit of chemistry. (Joe Pie Picture Library)

chemist shop and heated up in the tin in a saucepan of hot water. The resulting paste was spread onto a piece of linen or cotton sheeting, and while still hot, placed onto a patient's chest or back and kept there for days. It helped alleviate inflammation but anxious mothers often spread it onto the chest of their perfectly healthy children in the winter – just in case!

APERIENT. Medicines which produce a natural movement of the **bowels**. The weekly purge was part of life and **castor oil, flowers of sulphur, Gregory powder, prunes, rhubarb** products, **senna** and syrup of figs, **aloes, cascara,** were all used extensively adding to the sum of human misery. The rigours of the outside privy may have had something to do with the general constipation afflicting the population before the advent of indoor lavatories.

APHRODISIAC. A persistent urban myth held that those suffering from **tuberculosis** had a more rampant libido than was considered normal. This could be attributed to the fact you knew you were not going to live long and you might as well enjoy life. Women especially took on a wraith-like translucent beauty. However, it might just be that the middle classes had seen too many operas like *La Boheme* and *La Traviata*!

See also **liquorice, oatmeal, oysters** and **pussy willow**.

APOPLEXY. A sudden loss of consciousness often followed by paralysis caused by a rupture of a blood vessel in the brain; what we would now call a stroke. It was thought that anyone stout with a short neck and a florid complexion was most at risk.

In this instance the various recommendations in John Wesley's *Primitive Physic* could not have got it more wrong and would have been positively harmful.

'If the fit be soon after a meal, do not bleed, but vomit.'

'Rub the head, feet and hands strongly and let two strong men carry the patient upright, backwards and forwards about the room.'

'Drink quantities of pigeon's blood.'

The Wensleydale farmer Mr Brown recorded in his **commonplace book** in 1895: 'Recipe doctor recommended for G Weatherald after having a stroke. Into a jug put 1 pint of boiling water, 1 ounce of **Epsom salts**, 1 sliced lemon and a teaspoonful of Cream of Tartar. 1 wineglassful every morning before breakfast.' In other words something to keep the **bowels** working and a good example of how little could be done.

APOTHECARY. A well educated craftsman who would supply herbal remedies but also more exotic ingredients from abroad. Potions and ointments were made in his workshop and although apothecaries were mostly men, widows were allowed to carry on their husband's trade.

APPENDICITIS. It was seriously believed in my childhood that swallowing an apple pip would cause appendicitis.

APPETITE. From *The Family Physician* by Maximilian Hazlemore 1794. 'If want of appetite proceeds from errors in diet, or any other part of the patient's regime, it ought to be changed. If nausea and retchings shew that the stomach is loaded with crudities, a **vomit** will be of service. After this a gentle purge or two of **rhubarb**, or any of the bitter purging salts, may be taken. Though gentle evacuations be necessary, yet strong purges and vomits are to be avoided, as they weaken the stomach and hurt digestion.'

The disagreeable habit of making oneself sick was always a popular one for those fortunate enough in the past to have enough to eat. High class Romans certainly indulged in this so as to carry on eating vast amounts, as did certain French kings. However, by the 18th century it was recognised that powerful 'vomits' and 'purgings' were not the answer to an upset stomach.

APPLES. The benefit of fresh fruit was understood long before vitamin C was discovered. The Romans cultivated and used apples medicinally as a tonic and digestive stimulant. However, the luxury of an apple was not always available to the poor in towns. Apple 'scrumping', a kinder word than stealing, was a popular pastime for small boys and, if they were caught, led to many a thick ear.

'An apple a day keeps the doctor away' is good advice and was recommended by all the home remedy booklets. 'The free use of apples is a great assistant to brain work; children cannot use them too freely.' However, less helpful was the belief that applying rotten apples to the eyes helped cure 'dim sight'. See also **earache** and **stye**. A word of caution on the eating of apples. They are a cold fruit so eating too many or on a cold stomach, for example at breakfast, can lead to digestive upsets and a surfeit of wind!

ARNICA. A medicine derived from the plant *Arnica montana*.

Tincture of arnica is to be found in many home medicine cupboards as a valuable external treatment for sprains and bruises. Arnica relieves pain by its weak irritant action. See also **liniment**.

ARTHRITIS. Inflammation of a joint. Relief was had by rubbing on **arnica**. Another old remedy was warmed rock salt wrapped in a flannel and placed on the painful area.

Homemade rubbing **liniments** were made using **camphor**, **mustard** or **turpentine** and offered some temporary respite.

An old remedy for arthritis which is still popular today used **gin**. Empty a small box of sultanas into a container and pour over enough neat gin to cover. Let it stand until the sultanas have absorbed the gin and eat nine sultanas each day. Some have claimed that eating these gin-soaked sultanas has also had a good effect on the skin complaint psoriasis as well as their arthritis.

A cheap alternative to an expensive **spa** treatment was a daily hot bath with a handful of **Epsom salts** in the water.

ASH. A tree once believed to have magical properties which may explain John Wesley's advice in *Primitive Physic* for those frightened of snakes. 'The dew from the leaves of the Ash is good for snake bites, while a branch of the tree will prevent a snake coming near you.'

ASPARAGUS. Those who enjoy lightly steamed asparagus with a knob of butter should know that they are eating a food which has been around for 2,000 years. It was cultivated for its medicinal, restorative properties which include a cleansing action on the **bowels**, **liver** and kidneys.

ASTHMA. The narrowing of the bronchial tubes leading to difficulty in breathing. Also known in country areas as 'the risin' of the lights' as it was thought the lights (lungs) rose into the throat and stopped up the windpipe.

An 18th century cure was swallowing leaden bullets, the weight of which, it was believed, would keep down the lungs. Suggestions from John Wesley's *Primitive Physic* to relieve asthma were:

'Take a pint of cold water every night, as you lie down in bed.'

'A pint of cold water every morning, washing the head therein immediately after, and using the cold bath once a fortnight.'

'A spoonful of nettle juice, mixed with honey.'

'Live for a fortnight on boiled carrots only.'

'Wear a piece of moleskin on your chest.'

None of the above would have done you any harm although a diet of **carrots** is unwise, as in excessive amounts they can be toxic, giving the skin an orange glow. However, his further advice to 'Drink a pint of sea water every morning' is hard to stomach, as is 'Procure 7 spider webs, roll them up into a little ball and swallow them.'

The business with the carrots was still in favour in the 1930s as a *Housewife's Guide Book* recommended: 'Live chiefly on boiled carrots or leeks for a month; or drink a pint of new milk morning and evening.'

As asthma can be caused by allergies there may be some sense in having a restricted diet although many people are allergic to cows milk.

Within living memory anxious mothers made asthmatic children wear a small lump of **tar** round their neck believing it to help with breathing.

ASTHMATIC PERSONS. 'Those who are obliged to be in town all day ought, at least, to sleep out of it. Many asthmatic persons who cannot live in England, enjoy very good health in the south of France, Portugal, Spain or Italy.' Maximilian Hazlemore in 1794 advising foreign climes for the asthmatic.

Most people who suffered breathing difficulties did so because of the polluted atmosphere of industrial towns, lung diseases and general ill health rather than the asthma we know today. Sadly foreign travel and a second home were not an option for any other than the rich.

ATHLETE'S FOOT. The fungal infection *Tinea pedis* is a form of **ringworm** affecting the feet. Soaking the feet in your own **urine** was a fairly common remedy and one that was quite useful for keeping the feet clean.

B

Bottles of Liquor are followed by bottles of Physic.

BACKACHE. Hard manual labour and the winter elements meant an aching back at the end of the day. Farmer's wives heated an old fashioned flat iron in front of the fire, the farmer bent over and brown paper was placed onto his back. Very carefully the wife worked the iron over his back through the brown paper – wonderful firm heat that gave instant relief.

The dried leaves and flowering tops of the garden plant **golden rod** were, according to a 1930s home remedy book, 'used in the manner of tea' as a remedy for backache. It is a relaxant herb that reduces inflammation so was probably helpful.

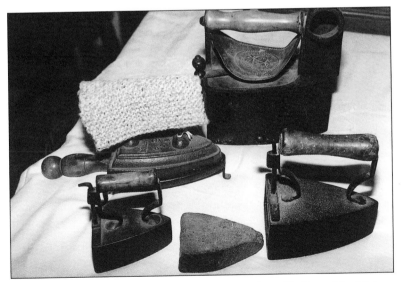

Unlikely aids for backache. These old flat irons were heated in front of the kitchen range and when hot the iron was pressed firmly onto brown paper laid on the painful part. As one iron cooled down you had another ready. (Photograph Ann Holubecki)

In his **commonplace book** dated 1895, Mr Edward Brown, a Yorkshire farmer, recorded a remedy that had worked for him: Quarter of an ounce each of oil of **juniper** and spirit of **lavender** and half an ounce each of spirit of **nitre** and **sal volatile**. 20 drops to be taken in half a wine glass of water 3 times a day.

BAD BREATH. An anti-social affliction that has at some time or other affected us all. In the past the likely cause was rotting teeth or gum disease but now more probably an excess of curry or garlic. An old trick was chewing **parsley** after a meal. Drinking **mint** tea or eating strawberries were all supposed to sweeten the breath.

BAD LEGS. A wide ranging term for a condition that could have been caused by any number of illnesses. As children in Cumbria we used to say we had a bone in our leg for a painful leg. A 1930s home remedy book listed Bad Legs in very vague terms: 'Bad Legs of long standing may be washed in **lime** water and milk daily, and to drink lime water and milk at the same time, good results may be expected.'

BAIRNING JOB. Yorkshire Dales dialect for a confinement which always took place in your own bed at home.

BALDNESS. Baldness is not really an illness but was always listed as such in old self-help books. The extraordinary sensitivity of some men about their receding hair-lines even now leads them into such style disasters and aberrations as combing a lock of hair from one side of the head to the other. So it is only right to include baldness here.

Boxwood, part of the *Cornus* or *Dogwood* species, appeared in several remedies. American boxwood (*Cornus florida*) has therapeutic properties which were used in the past for nervous exhaustion and tension headaches. Wash the head frequently with a **decoction** of boxwood.

A more inconvenient cure, according to John Wesley in his *Primitive Physic*, was rubbing the scalp morning and evening with an onion until it was red, followed by a further rubbing of **honey**. The drawback with this remedy was remaining confined to the house.

Nature provided several old cures; for example **nettle** juice combed through the hair.

Gather the stems of the wild thistle, put them through a mangle, collect and strain the liquid and bottle it. Rub on night and morning for 3 months and a 1920s home remedy book promised you would see a great change. Now it would be more difficult to find a mangle than the thistle.

An unusual remedy from Northamptonshire recommended rubbing pigeon droppings into the scalp.

BALSAM. A substance containing resins and benzoic acid. The most commonly used were Balsam of Peru, Balsam of Tolu and the all time favourite, even now – **friars' balsam**. They were used to relieve the symptoms of **coughs** and **colds**.

BARBER-SURGEON. Henry VIII granted a royal charter to the Barber-Surgeons Company in 1540. **Physicians** who were Oxford and Cambridge educated looked down their noses at barber-surgeons. They were craftsmen who passed on their limited surgical skills from father to son through a long apprenticeship. A red and white striped pole outside the shop advertised their skills in cutting and chopping.

Not known with any affection as 'Mr Sawbones', they were often quite burly characters as strength and a strong arm were needed in their line of work. They specialised in the rough end of medicine cutting out cysts, tumours and **bladder stones**, setting fractures, blood-letting, extracting teeth, draining pus and the occasional amputation – all the dirty bits of healthcare.

In 1745 the surgeons parted company with the barbers and from then on their prestige rose to unimaginable heights. The humble barber-surgeon of the 16th and 17th century would find it hard to imagine the almost 'god-like' status now attained by the surgeon.

BARLEY WATER. The medicinal uses of barley were first known by the Egyptians in 1550 BC. Women have always believed it to help with **cystitis**, an inflammation of the urinary bladder; barley is known to soothe irritated tissues.

It also aids digestion during convalescence, hence no hospital

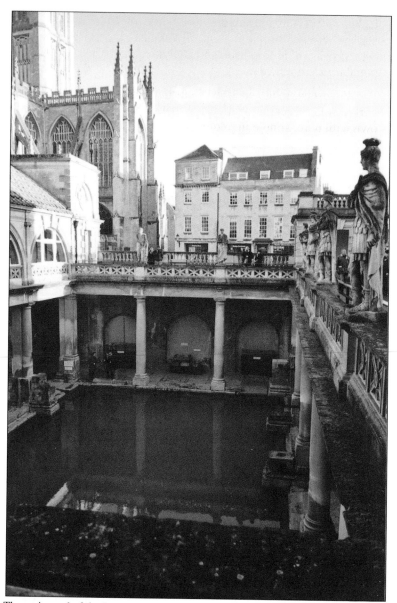

The main pool of the Roman Baths at Bath, now below modern street level. Bathing in the waters was said to 'Cleanse the body from all blotches, scurvical itchings and breakings out.'

locker in the past was without a bottle of Robinson's Lemon Barley Water. Matthias Robinson founded a medical remedies company in 1823, Robinson and Bellville, and barley water was a popular patent remedy.

The Victorians regarded it as a cure-all and until bottled lemon barley water became available in 1935 housewives made their own with pure, simple ingredients.

Mrs Hotchkin's Barley Water

Wash one tablespoon of Pearl Barley in different changes of water until the water runs clear. Strain and add the peel from a lemon but it must be very thin peel and not have any white pith attached. Sweeten with lump sugar and add the lemon juice then pour on 2 quarts of boiling water. Let it stand covered for one night then strain and bottle it. It will keep for 3 days.

BARRENNESS. The inability to produce children. A problem for all classes: royalty and the aristocracy needed heirs, the working class needed children to look after them in old age. In remote country areas, right up to the Second World War, it was quite acceptable to prove the woman fertile before marrying her. A wedding took place, if the woman was lucky, only after she had conceived.

For those needing help, fresh air, 'regulation of the **bowels**', **tonics** and **sea bathing** were all seen as an aid to pregnancy. A Doctor Taylor of Croydon in the mid 1800s put both husband and wife on a diet of milk and vegetables.

Certain foods were believed helpful in conceiving: **oysters**, fresh eggs, pigeons and lobsters.

A less pleasant option for the woman was **leeches** applied to the opening of the uterus.

BATH. It is claimed that the restorative properties of Bath's spring water were first discovered in 863 BC by a leper called Bladud, father of King Lear, who noticing his pigs were so much better after wallowing in a warm swamp, did the same and was cured of his **leprosy**. There are 43 minerals in the water including calcium and iron.

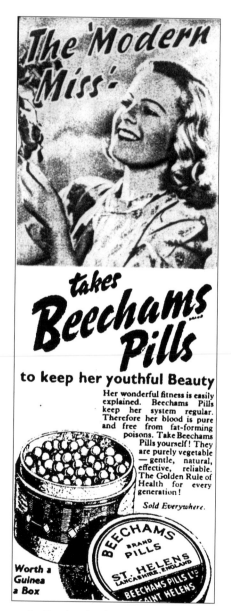

A 1939 advertisement for Beecham's Pills. The slogan 'Worth a guinea a box' became quite a catch phrase.

The natural hot springs of Aquae Sulis were sacred to the Romans and must have been a pleasing place to indulge in their favourite pastime of bathing. A magnificent Temple and Baths flourished from the 1st century AD but the significance of bathing was not something we British ever fully understood. When the Roman influence waned in the 5th century the baths were allowed to collapse and the stone work was quarried for other buildings.

The 12th century monks of Bath refurbished the spring as a medicinal bath claiming cures for paralysis, colic and **gout**. By the 16th and 17th centuries mixed bathing for medicinal and other less decorous purposes was very popular although Samuel Pepys, visiting in 1668 sounded a note of caution, 'Methinks it cannot be clean to go so many bodies together into the same water'. Indeed from our 21st century viewpoint if you had been quite well when you got into the water you had probably caught something by the time you got out.

Fashionable society flocked to Bath after Mary the wife of James II spent some time soaking in the waters and became pregnant. New ideas in the 17th century promoted drinking large quantities of the **spa** water and in 1706 the Pump Room was opened. A pint or two a day was recommended and in some extreme cases a gallon! Visitors were not pleased when a new Pump Room opened in 1795 with no provision for 'when the waters begin to operate'.

Dr Falconer of Bath believed firmly that there was no complaint for which Nature had not provided a suitable healing spring and the Bath waters cured everything from 'Cold Humours and Hypochondriacal Flatulence' to 'the Longing of Maids to eat Chalk, Coals and the Like'.

Bath is a beautiful, elegant city, for ever associated with Jane Austen, but as a spa town its days are past. Mixed bathing was forbidden in the early 19th century, the waters are only sipped in small doses by tourists in the Pump Room and you can no longer gaze down on the frolics and assignations taking place in the King's Bath.

BEECHAM'S PILLS. Thomas Beecham (1820–1907) founded the pharmaceutical firm – his grandson Sir Thomas Beecham became the world famous conductor. Beecham's Pills nicely catered for the Victorian obsession with their **bowels** as the early pills contained **aloes, ginger,** and **soap**, all purgatives. They were a favourite in the treatment of **biliousness, constipation, headache** and **indigestion**.

BEER. Seen as a safer alternative to **water**. Countrywomen made their own and workers were often given a ration a day. In the 19th century Black Country miners were entitled to 2 quarts of weak beer each day, the strength of the brew being a constant cause of complaint.

BEETROOT. The Romans used beetroot to relieve a **fever**. Current medical thinking recommends eating beetroot as a natural way to boost the immune system. Roast or boiled beetroot is rich in folate, which for women of childbearing age helps reduce the risk of spina bifida in babies. Beetroot wine was a popular homemade **tonic**.

BELCH. Drinking strong **tea** was thought to blame. See also **flatulence**.

BENJAMIN. Otherwise known as *Lindera benzoin* or spice bush and often included as an ingredient in old remedies just for good measure. Its chief claim to fame was a cure for **dysentery** and **worms**.

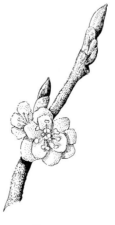

Benjamin

BENZOIC ACID. An antiseptic but also used internally for urinary infections.

BICARBONATE OF SODA. To be found in every kitchen cupboard as baking soda. A retired Sheffield fireman told me that in the late 1950s early 1960s they always carried a stone jar of bicarbonate of soda in the fire engine. When attending a fire where anyone was burned, they sprinkled the burn with the bicarb, wrapped a bandage round it and sprayed with water. He swore by the healing properties of bicarbonate of soda.

A teaspoon was added to the bathwater of a 'fractious baby'. A 1930s home remedy book advised, 'It has a wonderful effect in quieting the nervous irritation of a teething or otherwise cross child . . . it will go to sleep almost as soon as dried, and wake up as bright and amiable as one could desire.' See also **conception, heartburn, indigestion** and **teeth**.

BILIOUSNESS. A general term used when feeling unwell, irritable and possibly sick. The remedies offered in old home remedy books were consequently quite vague.

Drinking warm lemonade seemed to work miracles: 'this has cured when judged to be at the point of death'. Hot water drunk before breakfast was thought to cure a bilious attack; not dissimilar to the current craze for drinking at least 2 litres of water a day to cleanse the system of impurities. For those not able to manage all this liquid a teaspoonful of **blackcurrant** preserve before breakfast was just as good.

J. T. Butterworth in his *Practical Medical and Commercial Recipes* of 1897 offered words of advice relevant even today: 'The peculiar train of symptoms we term biliousness are merely a flag of warning which nature hangs out to tell the sufferer that his digestive organs reqire rest, and cannot go on smoothly again until they have had it. Hence it is that bilious people are forced to remain quiet and starve themselves until the attack has passed off.' See also **Beecham's Pills**.

BITTER ALOES. Children who persistently bit their nails had them painted with bitter aloes. The taste was awful and the shame of having the black painted nails was enough to make you stop.

BLACKBERRY. I have happy childhood memories of blackberry picking with my mother. An old blue enamel tin for collecting and a walking stick to pull down the brambles and then home to make jam or blackberry and apple pies. Do today's children scramble for brambles or is it considered too dangerous?

In past times the blackberry was believed to have mythical healing powers. For a cure sickly children and adults with **rheumatism** were passed through an arch of bramble that had rooted at both ends. A blackberry was never picked after the Old St Michaelmas Day, 11th October as country people believed Satan had urinated on it! Folklore said that when Satan was cast out of Paradise he fell into a bramble bush and on every anniversary of the Fall, he either spits or pees on the blackberries.

The leaves are astringent and when made into a vinegar soothed a **sore throat** or **tonsillitis**.

Blackberry Vinegar

Put 1 pint each of blackberries and white wine vinegar in a large screw top jar for a week, shaking the jar several times a day. Strain into a saucepan and add 1 lb of sugar and 8 ounces of **honey** and bring to the boil. When sugar and honey are dissolved, allow to cool and bottle. Take a tablespoonful in a glass of hot water at bedtime.

A strong **infusion** of blackberry leaves was believed to relieve **shingles**.

BLACKCURRANTS. These were once named quinsy berries as they were thought effective in relieving **quinsy**. An astringent tonic herb that reduces inflammation, fresh blackcurrants are very high in vitamin C. In the 18th and 19th centuries blackcurrant leaves, which contain tannins, were used to supplement tea leaves when there was a shortage or the price too high. Blackcurrant tea in Victorian times was drunk for 'disordered bowels'.

A teaspoon of blackcurrant jam in hot water was a cure for **colds** and **sore throats**.

An old Cumbrian recipe for a **sore throat**.

Blackcurrant Vinegar

Boil a quart of fully ripe blackcurrants and a good bunch of currant leaves until tender. Squeeze through a jelly bag. For every quart of juice add 24 ounces of sugar and 30 fluid ounces of **vinegar**. Boil for 30 minutes. A small glass of spirits will add a little 'kick' to this vinegar.

BLACK DEATH. A terrible disease which spread across Europe from Asia in the middle of the 14th century killing an estimated 25 million Europeans. It arrived in the ports of Bristol and Weymouth in 1348 via rats unwittingly transported in ships and swept through Exeter, Bridgewater, Bath, Winchester, Oxford, London and into West Kent and then northwards to York and on into Scotland. Villages were decimated and often rebuilt away from the original infection. To this day fields and place names reflect where the dead were buried.

The infected fleas from rats with the disease *Yersinia pestis* bit humans resulting in swollen lymph nodes in the groin, neck or armpits. The pus-filled swelling or bubo, from which we get the other name of **bubonic plague**, turned black due to haemorrhaging under the skin and burst. Delirium and death were not far away. Pneumonic plague developed from bubonic plague and spread quickly on the breath and clothes. The lungs became choked with an evil smelling sputum and death from septicaemia came as a blessing.

William Dene, a monastic writer, wrote of West Kent, 'The mortality was so great that none could be found to carry the corpses to the grave. Men and women bore their offspring on their shoulders to the church, and cast them into a common pit. From these there came so great a stench that hardly anyone dared to cross the cemetery.'

So many clergy died that the Church took the pragmatic decision in 1349 for the sick to confess their sins to a layman or **even a woman**!

BLACKHEADS. Eruptions of little black spots indicating the sebaceous duct is choked with dirt and sebum. *The Lady's World* of 1898 advised; 'Blackheads or Comedones – empty the blackheads of their contents by pressing firmly over them with the end of a watch-key. This should be done daily.'

BLADDER STONES. These were very common, perhaps because of all the impurities in what was drunk. A Somerset doctor wrote to the *British Medical Journal* in 1872 that in Frome, Somerset bladder stones were rarely seen and he was of the opinion that the **beer** and cider drunk by the local men was a preventative measure. In response to this a Newcastle doctor felt that the frequency of bladder stones in Northumberland and Durham was entirely due to the drinking water containing **lime** and magnesia. The first doctor wondered if Northern men ever drank anything other than water – which he thought very unlikely and advised them to change to beer.

Up to the 19th century the removal of a bladder stone was often carried out by a **barber surgeon**, who could wield a knife as well as anyone. It was quite common to call in unqualified 'specialists' if you wanted something done medically. Itinerant tooth drawers and those who would operate on a cataract plus roving lithotomists who removed bladder stones were all available at a price.

Bladder stones may be up to the size of a goose egg and in the past there was no real option but to have them surgically removed. Many claimed they could dissolve the stone in the bladder without the need to resort to the travelling lithotomist and it must have been tempting to try. Drinking the water in which parsnips had been boiled, dried kidney beans burnt to a powder and then used as tea and eating a slice of dried bread every morning were just some of the remedies tried. In 1739 a secret recipe known only to a Mrs Joanna Stephens was thought to be so effective that the British Government bought the secret from her for the huge amount of £5,000. It turned out to consist of roasted egg shells, **soap** and aromatic bitters.

BLISTER. A swelling caused by an accumulation of clear fluid under the skin and most commonly found on the feet where shoes rubbed. In many poor families shoes were handed down after a child had grown out of them, so you were unlikely ever to have a pair that fitted exactly.

An easy remedy was a paste made from **soap** and water.

However to relieve a blister – and I have seen this done by long distance walkers – take a needle and cotton and pass it through the blister, leaving a length of cotton on either side. The contents will seep out into the thread. See also **urine**.

BLISTER, TO. Apply a counter irritant producing small blisters. A popular method for dealing with practically any illness, including **post natal depression**, where it was unlikely to have lifted the spirits. It was based on the principle of relieving congestion deep within the body. **Mustard** and **turpentine** were both used for blistering but the effects were slightly mitigated by spreading them on a cloth or **brown paper** which was then placed on the body. **Cantharides** and **iodine** were both painted directly onto the skin.

BLOOD-LETTING. Much in vogue for centuries, blood-letting or bleeding was the medical profession's answer to everything. Even if you were not ill, people believed that if you were bled regularly you avoided bad health. It was something of a springtime ritual and seen as a tonic. **Cupping, leeches** and **scarification** were all methods used but the most common was to tie a bandage round the arm to make the veins in the forearm swell up and then open the vein with a knife. You could demand a blood-letting by a **barber-surgeon** or avail yourself of the services of a local **apothecary** as in Knaresborough, Yorkshire, where you sat in the shop on a red leather couch to be bled. Often people were not happy until they had fainted with loss of blood and many died, not of their illness, but of excessive bleeding. Even Mrs Beeton in her *Book of Household Management* of 1861 gave instructions on how to bleed oneself in an emergency!

BLOOD, TO RENEW. After undergoing the ritual of **blood-letting** the next step was purifying the blood and it was the principal treatment for many illnesses. This recipe from a 1920s home remedy book was easily prepared from ingredients in the kitchen cupboard: 'A Recipe Invaluable – The simplest and best blood purifier known is a sliced **lemon**, 2 tablespoons of **blackcurrant** preserve and 10 red **sage** leaves to a quart of boiling water, sweetened to taste, which makes a most agreeable drink.'

Commonly used and of real nutritional value, **watercress** was a **spring tonic** for ordinary people. The 'quickest renewer of blood is to boil watercress for ten minutes and drink the water in milk'. We would make a delicious watercress soup now. **Burdock** was considered to be one of the finest blood purifyers.

General malaise was often attributed to 'impure blood'. A common remedy to improve the blood was to dissolve 2 ounces of **Epsom salts**, 3 lemons, 2 ounces of cream of tartar and half an ounce of ground **ginger** in a quart of **hop** tea and drink a glass while fasting. Another example of treating the body to the all too familiar purge.

BOILS. Most young men until recently expected an outbreak of boils on the back of the neck; the starched collar was to blame. Given that up to the 1950s men wore a collar and tie on all occasions whether at work or play – I have a family photograph of father on Margate beach in trilby hat, full three piece suit, collar and tie – the chafing caused by excessive starching of collars would have caused major skin irritation. Bacteria thrived on a dirty sweaty collar and the germs lived happily in the hair follicle bursting into activity just when you wanted to look your best.

Women dealt with the unpleasant business of men's boils. There were various treatments and most involved pain with extreme heat applied to the boil, often in the form of a **poultice**. This could be made from heated **bread**, **honey** mixed with a little flour, **linseed**, **oatmeal**, a **soap** and sugar paste or hot mashed **turnips**.

The excruciating 'milk-bottle treatment' involved pouring boiling water into a glass milk bottle, emptying the water out and placing the steam filled bottle over the boil, holding it there while it cooled and the pus was drawn out. The pain was intense and sometimes the suction so great that you had to get a hammer to break the bottle!

Hot fomentations were prepared but an easier way was a cooked jacket potato in a stocking held onto the boil.

Other forms of heat applied to the boil depended on where the boil was situated. One on the bottom meant sitting on a chamber pot containing very hot water mixed with **Epsom salts**. Also

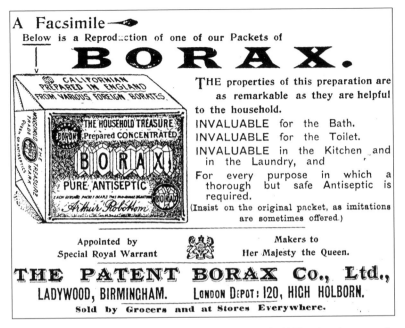

Borax was an invaluable part of Victorian life in the early 1900s when it was used as a household antiseptic. From *The Lady's World* 1899.

involving the chamber pot but this time the contents; drinking one's **urine** was seen as a cure for boils, though I have never met anyone prepared to admit doing this.

If in doubt attack the boil from inside with a good purge. An old early 1900s **commonplace book** advised: 'Boil 1 pound of figs and 4 ounces of **figwort** in 2 quarts of water for 30 minutes. Drink a wineglass of this 3 times a day adding as much **saltpetre** as will go on a threepenny bit.'

From Wiltshire another old internal remedy advised a small amount of fresh **yeast** mixed with a small glass of fresh water drunk directly after breakfast.

An old country remedy used extensively and very successfully was a fresh cowpat wrapped in gauze and placed on the boil to 'draw' it. No wonder elderly men still bear the scars of this home treatment!

BORAX. At one time found in every bathroom cupboard and used in a solution to calm itching and chapped skin; now we are advised not to use it on babies and young children. Borax was also an effective **dandruff** treatment before medicated shampoos. Its beneficial properties were not just useful for the skin but as a household cleaner and a 1930s home remedy book advised, 'Spiders will not come where shelves are washed with borax.'

BOWELS. For centuries keeping regular was synonymous with good health and the nation's bowels took a hammering. In any illness the first course of action was to attend to the bowels. Dire warnings were to be found in every journal as to the consequences of a costive habit. Victorian women were accused of being particularly prone to 'neglecting to solicit a periodical evacuation of the bowels'.

J. T. Butterworth in his *Practical Medical and Commercial Recipes* of 1897 spoke for the entire medical profession when he wrote, 'It is a cardinal rule that the bowels should act once in every 24 hours.' To achieve this perfection of habit vast quantities of **aperients** and **purgatives** were regularly taken.

BRAN. As a medium for retaining heat a bran **poultice** applied to a painful area gave soothing relief. Also useful in the healing process, a handful of bran boiled in water, strained and cooled and the liquid used to bathe an ulcerated **leg**.

BREAD. This staple commodity known as 'the staff of life' was usually available, even if little other food was to be found, in the cupboards of the poor. If you were hungry you ate bread to fill up and bread and jam was eaten as a snack between meals.

Bread and **honey** was a simple remedy for insomnia and eaten for supper gave a good night's sleep. I have not recommended any remedies in this book but something like this would do no harm and might even help those who long for a good night's sleep. See also **sleeplessness**.

Toasted bread held against the ear relieved **earache,** and for a **sore throat**, burnt toast was soaked in vinegar, warmed and placed inside a stocking round the throat.

BREAD POULTICE. Everyone in the past believed in the efficacy of the bread poultice. Used as a cure for a **boil**, **whitlow** and **abscess** until the 1950s and also extensively in the treatment of **pneumonia**. The application of a bread poultice was unlikely to effect a cure for pneumonia but the heat might relieve the pain felt on coughing or drawing breath.

How the poultice was made varied from family to family but in general the method was as follows: Place stale breadcrumbs in a basin, pour enough boiling water over the crumbs to soak them. Allow to cool slightly; drain off the excess liquid and spread between two pieces of cloth; place poultice onto affected area. Modern medicine has relegated this everyday knowledge to a book such as this one.

BREASTS. One of the few advantages of dying young in the past was that diseases familiar to us now were less common; we did not live long enough for them to develop. Breast cancer is an example, its seriousness recognised and crude attempts at surgery made even in the 18th century. Mastectomy operations took place, such as the one described by the novelist Fanny Burney, who underwent an operation for cancer of the breast in 1810 and amazingly lived to write of her excrutiating agony while under the knife without anaesthetic: 'When the dreadful steel was plunged into the breast – cutting through veins – arteries – flesh – nerves – I needed no injunctions not to restrain my cries. I began a scream that lasted unintermittingly during the whole time of the incision. . .'

Breasts can be a nuisance: women suffer inflammation and an abscess, often as a result of a cracked nipple while breast feeding and discomfort just before and at the start of the monthly period.

Women's inventiveness knew no bounds. From Northwich in Cheshire I learned that an uncooked **cabbage** leaf placed in the bra when breastfeeding prevented nipple soreness and from Sheffield that women once applied a cowpat wrapped in gauze to the breast to heal an **abscess**. For unspecified breast pain quantities of **laudanum** were drunk to deaden the pain.

For 'Hard Breasts' John Wesley in his *Primitive Physic* put his trust in **turnips** and advised applying mashed roast turnip mixed with a little oil of roses and keeping the breast very warm with a flannel.

For 'Soft breasts and swell'd; boil a handful each of **chamomile** and mallow (**marshmallow**) in milk and water and forment (*sic*) with it between two flannels as hot as can be borne every 12 hours. It also dissolves any Knob or swelling in any part.' Heat seems to have been the chief comforter in all this.

Advances in medicine mean that breast problems are successfully treated. What would women coping with pain and discomfort in the past make of the 21st century need for perfect silicone breasts? Today large sums of money are spent willingly to go under the knife for a spot of surgical enhancing or reducing. Women in the past would have settled for being comfortable.

BRIGHTON. See **sea bathing** and **sea water**.

BRIMSTONE. An old name for **sulphur**.

BRONCHITIS. From the 18th century onwards if you lived in an industrial town you expected a dose of bronchitis every winter. Smoke, soot and pollution poured from factory chimneys, furnaces and coal fires. General health was so bad that for many a bad **cough** and congestion of the **lungs** were part of a short, miserable life. Unknowingly even the addictive pleasure of cigarette smoking added to the sum of this misery. Bad housing and large families in cramped and damp conditions in a cold, wet, foggy climate all resulted in unhealthy diseased **lungs**.

The general medical advice to not sleep in the same underclothing as worn during the day and to wear a wash leather constantly on the chest was singularly ineffective. Vast quantities of **cough medicines** were made at home. See also **antimony**, **goose grease** and **tar**.

BROOM. *Cytisus scoparius*. All parts of this plant are highly poisonous with powerful narcotic properties. It was once used to treat a failing heart.

In the West Midlands 'broom tea' was prepared by pouring boiling water over the flowers and leaving it to cool; the resulting liquid

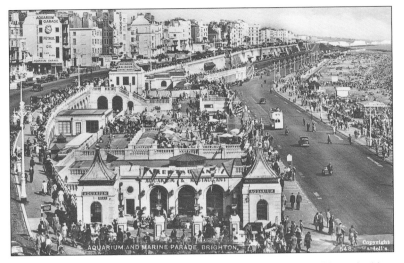

A postcard of prewar Brighton by A. Wardell. No longer a fashionable sea bathing resort but now an easy journey by train for Londoners to enjoy a day out. My mother always maintained that if you were poorly, 'A day in Brighton is worth a week anywhere else.'

was said to purify the blood. Word of mouth must have advised what quantities to use when making this highly dangerous tea. However, the 'tea' also had a powerful purging action and with this always came a belief that it must be doing some good.

BROWN PAPER. There was always some handy to wrap parcels and you never threw any away. Even today there are some who hoard brown paper and string! Brown paper was worn under the vest or liberty bodice to keep in body heat. However, first the chest was rubbed with either **camphor**, **goose grease** or **turpentine** and sometimes a mixture of all three!

BRUISE. Otherwise known as a contusion it is the outward sign of bleeding in the deeper parts of the skin and underlying tissue, as a result of an injury or knock. Bruises are colourful going from black and blue to brown and finally yellow. A cold compress or an astringent substance like **witch hazel** can help to prevent more bleeding.

John Wesley in *Primitive Physic* understood this, 'Immediately apply a cloth, 5 or 6 times doubled, dipt in cold water, and new dipt when it grows warm.'

His less pleasant ideas involved an application of animal dung. From the same book he advised a treacle and **brown paper** plaster and 200 years later this was still being recommended in the home remedy books of the 1930s.

In Warwickshire they used **sage** leaves and in the West Country **marshmallow** leaves mixed with pig's fat.

My mother favoured a knob of butter and a penny tied onto the bruise.

BUBONIC PLAGUE. Over the centuries outbreaks of Bubonic Plague, or the **Black Death** as it was known in the Middle Ages, continued to erupt across the world and this country. The one remembered from school history lessons is always The Great Plague of London which lasted from 1665 to the summer of 1666 and killed an estimated 100,000 people. Samuel Pepys recorded in his diary on the 30th April 1665, 'Great fears of the sicknesse here in the City, it being said that two or three houses are already shut up. God preserve us all.' Later he wrote of not daring to wear his new periwig, 'Because the plague was in Westminster when I bought it. And it is a wonder what will be the fashion after the plague is done as to periwigs, for nobody will dare to buy any haire for fear of the infection – that it had been cut off of the heads of people dead of the plague.'

Wealthy people shut up their houses and fled. Pepys packed his wife Elizabeth off to the safety of Woolwich and wrote his will. Fashionable city women put their faith in sweet smelling pomanders and men thought tobacco smoke would ward off infection. The disease spread and some isolated communities like **Eyam** in Derbyshire realised that they must cut themselves off from others to contain the disease.

Desperate people clutched at increasingly bizarre remedies: a warm pigeon or chicken with plucked tail feathers held against the swelling, a mastiff puppy held to the breast and live frogs placed on the sore.

The nursery rhyme *Ring-a-ring o' roses* described the symptons of the plague but the second, less well known verse 'Down in the meadow eating buttercups – Atishoo, atishoo, we all stand up' may refer to eating the flowers and juice of the **marigold** which many thought beneficial. Large quantities of poisonous ivy berries were used, with some success, to increase perspiration in the hope of sweating the sickness out.

BURDOCK. *Arctium lappa*. As a child one of my favourite drinks was fizzy **dandelion** and burdock, known affectionately as 'dandy-burd'. For centuries burdock was used in the treatment of an impressive list of diseases: **convulsions**, digestive problems, **eczema**, **jaundice**, **kidney** disease, **leprosy**, **scrofula**, **scurvy**, **ulcers**, **venereal disease** and on top of all these the plant was thought to be an excellent purifier of the **blood**. There must have been some truth in this as even now it is valued as a herb that reduces inflammation and controls bacterial infection. The root, stem and leaves of burdock can be boiled or eaten raw.

BURNS. For superficial burns and **scalds** current medical thinking advises pouring cold water onto the affected area for at least 10 minutes. John Wesley in his *Primitive Physic* was on the right track when he advised in 1747, 'plunge the part into cold water;

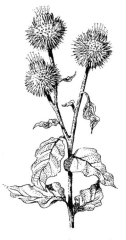

Lesser Burdock

keep it in an hour if not well before.' However, that wisdom was lost for, until recently, we believed in slathering substantial amounts of butter or **olive oil** onto a burn, which had the effect of further frying the skin!

Keeping the air off the burn was the aim of all the old remedies and to that end interesting substances were applied: a paste of flour and cold water, a **poultice** of oatmeal and cold water, **bicarbonate of soda**, a layer of **Carron oil** and cotton wool, an **onion**, a mixture of oil and **parsley**, or oil and **ginger**, cold **tea** leaves, a slice of raw potato or a nice gentle smearing of **honey**. See also **wounds**.

BUXTON. The Romans first discovered the value of Buxton's mineral waters and fresh air. In 1570 a Dr Jones in *The Benefit of the Auncient Bathes of Buckstones* claimed that the **spa** water was superior to that of **Bath**. Indeed the natural mineral water is without the unpleasant sulphur smell usually associated with **spa** cures. To take the waters you were subject to a means test: a yeoman paid 1 shilling, a duke 3 pounds 10 shillings and an archbishop 5 pounds. (Sadly current remuneration in the Church has not kept pace!)

The waters were considered more than medicinal, verging on the miraculous and Dr Jones expected his bathers to pray on entering the water. Belief in the powers of the water did not diminish and Holy **wells** are still venerated in Derbyshire in the annual 'well-dressing' ceremonies.

BYSSINOSIS. A thickening of the lung tissue caused by breathing in cotton dust. Once known as brown lung disease or Monday fever as it became worse on a Monday after a weekend away from the dust. It was most common among the workers in the Lancashire cotton mills. The symptoms are very like **bronchitis** and were treated with the same remedies. The ideal cure of removing oneself from the cause was not open to the working class poor.

C

There is a doctor in every hedge.

CABBAGE. Cabbage is forever linked with the smell of school corridors; the stale aroma of cooked cabbage and unwashed pubescent bodies. Once known as 'the medicine of the poor', cabbage was used for centuries in the treatment of skin conditions and chest infections. It is highly nutritious when eaten raw although, as a nation, we are determined to have our cabbage well cooked, thus destroying the vitamin C.

Holding a **rheumatic** joint over the steam from the saucepan while cooking cabbage is said to relieve pain, although care should be taken when trying this, or see **scalds**. A safer method was a hot **poultice** of cabbage leaves.

The outer leaf of a cabbage placed inside a hat will keep the head cool and inside a bra will prevent sore nipples in nursing mothers.

Eat raw cabbage leaves to prevent drunkenness.

CALF'S FOOT JELLY. Every Victorian novelist obliged the heroine to visit the poor and the sick with a bowl of this jelly, considered to be highly nourishing and suitable for invalids. Like most of my generation I have never made it – but on turning to my mother's *Enquire Within Upon Everything* given to her in 1930, I learned it required me to 'Slit the foot in two and take away every bit of fat off the claws . . . boil gently for 7 hours' – I never shall.

CAMPHOR. This was sold for home use in small squares or as oil. It is a solid, crystalline, oily substance distilled from the wood of a species of laurel. At one time camphor was found in every house in England, even if just in the wardrobe to deter moths and fleas – but no longer. Camphor's powerful properties have been recognised and an excess can cause poisoning and even death. Any pharmacist would advise extreme caution in using it, which will come as a surprise to readers who grew up smelling and using camphor regularly.

Camphor lockets were worn round the neck by children in winter to ward off childhood illnesses, camphor and water snuffed up the nose helped a **cold** and taken internally with a little water was thought to cure **sciatica**. See also **vampers**.

CAMPHORATED OIL. Often mixed with **goose grease** to make a powerful and pungent chest and back rub. Camphor was so much part of childhood that in the playground we would sing to the tune of *John Brown's Body*:

> John Brown's baby's got a cold upon its chest,
> John Brown's baby's got a cold upon its chest,
> John Brown's baby's got a cold upon its chest –
> And they rubbed it with camphorated oil.
> Cam-phor-am-phor-am-phor-aaaated.
> Cam-phor-am-phor-am-phor-aaaated
> Cam-phor-am-phor-am-phor-aaaated -
> And they rubbed it with camphorated oil!

CANCER. This is an ancient disease and one which the Greek physician Hippocrates (c460-c357 BC) named *karcinos* the Greek word for crab, perhaps describing the pain of a pinch from a crab claw. In the medieval world cancer was thought to be caused by an imbalance of the **humours** with too much black bile. The disease was rarely mentioned and although we cannot know for sure, one reason certainly in the past was that relatively few people lived into old age when cancers are most common.

Many of the illnesses diagnosed in the past, for example severe **dyspepsia**, may in reality have been cancer of the stomach. Extreme cases of **constipation** may have been cancer of the bowel; we will never know.

The word cancer was not to be found in family **commonplace books** or home remedy publications. Perhaps the taboo surrounding the illness was too great to see it written in such intimate everyday books. However, there was certainly an urban myth which believed that certain people had a 'cancer personality'. These people supposedly 'bottled things up' and swallowed their anger.

CANTHARIDES. A powder, sometimes known as Spanish Fly, made from the dried bodies of the Southern European beetle,

Cantharis vesicatoria. It was popular, at least with the medical profession, as an extremely painful blistering agent. See **blister**.

CARBUNCLE. A spreading collection of **boils** and treated in the same way. Called Rosy Drop if the carbuncle was on the face.

CARMINATIVE. A substance able to relieve **flatulence**. **Ginger** and **peppermint** were the most popular of those used, especially in patent medicines.

CARRON OIL. A patent medicine in the 1920s for treating **burns**. Made of equal parts **linseed** or **olive oil** and **lime** water it was spread onto a burn. It fell from favour in the 1930s when medical opinion changed and oil on a burn was seen as a bad thing.

CARROTS. Mothers encouraged childen to eat their carrots, saying it would make them see in the dark. Like so many 'old wives tales' there was an element of truth. Night-blindness is thought to be caused in some cases by vitamin A deficiency and the vegetable rich in this vitamin is the humble carrot.

CASCARA SAGRADA. The extract from the bark of a Californian tree and once used as a powerful **purgative**.

CASTOR OIL. The remembered joys of the weekly dose! A thick colourless oil from the seeds of the tropical castor-oil plant, *Ricinus communis* used extensively as a favourite **purgative** and also in some homemade **cough medicines**. After taking this who would dare to cough! See also **warts**.

CATAPLASM. An old word for **poultice**. In the early 1800s cataplasms of fresh cow dung were recommended for **bruises**.

CAYENNE. A 1930s home remedy book felt so strongly about cayenne that this advice appeared in capital letters: 'ITS PROPERTIES WORTH BETTER ACQUAINTANCE – Cayenne is the purest and strongest stimulant, and comes nearest to an universal remedy for almost any complaint, from the fact that it quickens the vital force to throw off any disease.'

Cayenne was a vital ingredient in **medical botany** in the 1800s. It was taken in a cupful of boiling water, allowed to stand for twenty minutes, the water poured from the grounds into another cup and drunk. The taste was such that anyone drinking it deserved to get better! See also **cough medicines**.

CELANDINE. *Chelidonium majus*, also known as the greater celandine or swallow wort and not related to the lesser celandine. See **pilewort**. Swallow oil was made commercially and it was named 'swallow' because the plant comes into flower when the swallows arrive and dies back when they leave. Swallows are said to pluck the flower to feed to their young, who are born blind, which might explain why an old Somerset cure for eye troubles used the juice from the stalk. However, the celandine has potentially dangerous properties which can effect breathing. See also **Zambuk**.

CHALICE WELL. See also **wells**. The Chalice Well on the slope of the Tor at Glastonbury in Somerset was at one time probably the most famous chalybeate spring in England. It is reputed to be the place where Joseph of Arimathea buried the chalice used at the Last Supper. Glastonbury waters were claimed to have curative properties for such diverse illnesses as **asthma, deafness, dropsy, leprosy, scrofula** and **ulcers**. For a few short years people flocked there to drink the water and at the height of its fame in the middle of the 1700s as many as 10,000 people were said to have visited in one month.

CHAMOMILE. Alternative spelling camomile *Chamaemelum nobile*. It was once widely cultivated for medicinal purposes. Chamomile flower tea was recommended for **heartburn**, nausea, painful menstruation and as a sedative. Chamomile is known as 'the plant's physician' as poor specimens thrive if it is planted alongside. Blondes also use a rinse of chamomile flowers to lighten the hair. See also **wind**.

CHANGE OF LIFE. A euphemism for the menopause. Hot flushes, night sweats, depression, insomnia, fatigue, anxiety, headaches, abnormal periods – you name it the menopause can throw it at you. In the 18th century **blood-letting** was supposed to relieve any unpleasant symptoms, although one doubts it.

Menopausal women were offered little advice except for a dose of **senna** occasionally, as the bowels were to be carefully regulated during this difficult time. A 1920s home remedy book went further: 'Keep the bowels open, take very little alcohol, have warm baths. Husbands should exercise great patience during this irritable period.'

For night sweats a hot salt bath was recommended, followed by a rub with a rough towel and a cup of cold **sage** tea.

See also **Sarsaparilla**

CHAPPED HANDS. The weekly washing and wringing of clothes for a large family by hand, often in cold wash houses meant sore chapped hands. It was said that rinsing the hands in potato water helped. **Mutton suet** and hog's lard were all rubbed on as hand cream. In the Black Country they used **honey** for all cracked and sore hands.

In farming families an old jar was kept in the kitchen containing a mixture of lard and **goose grease** and hands were dipped in the jar before going out to work in the wind and frost.

An old farmhouse recipe used 4 ounces of softened lard mixed with a little rosewater, 2 egg yolks and a big spoonful of **honey** and a little **oatmeal**. This was made into a paste and spread on the hands overnight and you went to bed wearing cotton gloves to keep the mixture on. See also **Snowfire ointment**.

CHAPPED LIPS. See also **chapped hands**. An old farmer rode into market and on dismounting from his horse went round to the back and kissed the horse's bottom. The other farmers asked in horror, 'What did you do that for?' The farmer replied, 'I've got chapped lips.' The others asked, 'Does that make them better then?' The old farmer replied, 'No, but it certainly stops me licking them!'

CHELTENHAM. Once a small Cotswold village where in 1718 a mineral spring was discovered by observing that the local pigeons flocked to peck at the mineral deposits. (A pigeon still appears on the town's coat of arms.) In 1738 the first Pump Room was built and 50 years later George III (1738–1820) gave Cheltenham his seal of approval by visiting to try and cure his 'madness'. He suffered from the disease porphyria, which was not understood

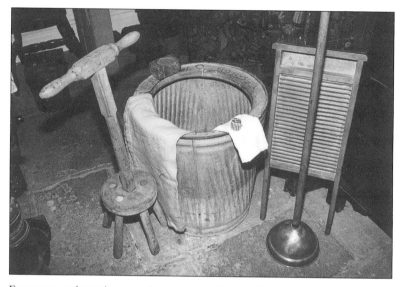

For women at home housework was hard and heavy. These were your washday appliances: a dolly tub, posser, washboard, soap and a Reckitt's Blue bag. By the end of the day your hands were chapped, cracked and sore. (Photograph Ann Holubecki)

and indeed the newspapers of the day at one time, rather unfairly, blamed the water of Cheltenham for his disorder.

The mineral waters were thought to be particularly good for **jaundice** in those returning from the Colonies, presumably suffering from **malaria**. The town was rebuilt between 1800 and 1840 at the height of the popularity of **spa** treatments, a fine example of a Georgian town built for people of taste and discernment.

CHICKEN SOUP. Known as Jewish penicillin. Hot and spicy foods have been scientifically proved to alleviate flu-like viruses and promote mucous secretions. However, the smell alone of homemade chicken soup would lift the spirits and tempt a jaded appetite.

CHILBLAINS. The itching and inflammation of chilblains is caused by poor circulation and cold. It was a common problem, judging from the rich variety of remedies.

The unlikely old cure of a brisk walk barefoot in the snow would only partly do you good. Standing in snow and then going inside and rubbing the feet briskly with a rough towel might have pepped up the circulation.

Others preferred patent medicines such as **Snowfire ointment**. Kitchen cupboard items were on hand to rub on the chilblain with, I should imagine, mixed success:

A sliced **onion** dipped in salt.
A mixture of **mustard** powder and brandy.
Hot roasted **turnips**.
The juice of a leek mixed with cream.
Wash the feet in water in which unpeeled potatoes have been boiled and if all else fails soak the feet in **urine** from the chamber pot.
A mixture of **mustard** and lard after first washing the feet in hot water in which washing soda had been dissolved.
Thrash the chilblain with a branch of holly!

CHILDBIRTH. Until recently always a risky business. It was known for centuries in what position a baby should be in the womb for a safe delivery. Knowing and achieving that position were two different things and many women died in childbirth. A woman was attended by female family and friends with perhaps the additional intervention of a midwife, not all of whom were women. In the 18th century the stronger arm of the new men-midwives or accoucheurs developed some skill with forceps in difficult births.

These midwives were a mixed blessing as the need for strict cleanliness and antiseptic procedures were unknown. Even if a woman was safely delivered she was likely to die shortly after from **puerperal fever**, a mostly streptococcal infection.

Opium–based drinks were given to dull the pain of childbirth but it was not until Queen Victoria was given chloroform during the birth of Prince Leopold in 1853 that it became acceptable for women to be given some pain relief. Indeed prior to Her Majesty leading the way the male medical view of childbirth can be summed up by Thomas J. Graham MD writing in his *On the*

Diseases of Females in 1841: 'In everything which relates to the act of parturition, Nature, not disturbed by disease, or molested by interruption, is fully competent to accomplish her own purpose; she may be truly said to disdain and to abhor assistance. Instead therefore of despairing and thinking they are abandoned in the hour of their distress, all women should believe and find comfort in the reflection, that they are at those times under the peculiar care of Providence.'

In John Wesley's *Primitive Physic*: 'To Cause an early Delivery – Fry sliced onion, 'till it is tender, boil this with half a glass of water; Strain and drink it in the morning fasting, for two or three weeks before the time of Child-birth.'

Drinking **raspberry** leaf tea in the final stages of pregnancy was said to ease childbirth as the herb tones the uterine muscles.

After the birth women in country areas might have their legs tied together for up to 10 days to prevent a haemorrhage.

CHILDCARE. Today everyone is an expert with books, articles and earnest academic papers on how to bring an adorable baby through the infections, allergies and tantrums of those early years. In the past our older female relatives told us what to do. A simple diet was always considered best with plenty of milk and porridge.

John Wesley in his *Primitive Physic* had some unusual advice: 'Wife parents should dip their children in cold water every morning, 'till they are three quarters old; and afterwards their Hands and Feet. No child should be swath'd tight. It lays the foundation for many diseases – 'Tis best to wean a child at about seven months old. No wife parent should suffer a child to drink any **tea**; (or at least, 'till it is ten or twelve years old) or to taste Spice or Sugar. Milk, Milk-porridge and Water-gruel are the proper Breakfast for Children. Washing the Head every morning in cold water, prevents **rheums**, and cures Coughs, Old Headachs and Sore Eyes.'

For a child who was out of sorts a teaspoonful of dill water or **lime** water mixed with milk soothed or if all else failed a mild purgative dose of **Turkey rhubarb** to clear the **bowels**.

Most households preferred and believed that children should be seen and not heard.

CHIN COUGH. An old word for **whooping cough**.

CHLORODYNE. Most commonly associated with Dr John Collis Browne, the physician who had first used it while serving with the Army in India. In 1854, while on leave, he was asked to go to Trimdon in County Durham to help with an outbreak of cholera. His medicine, which he called 'chlorodyne', was fairly successful and became one of the most popular patent remedies of the late 19th and early 20th centuries.

The ingredients were the highly addictive chloroform and morphine and many became unhappy with its widespread use. Chlorodyne was the main ingredient in many remedies for **coughs** and **colds**. A tuppenny bottle from the chemist of chlorodyne mixed with **liquorice** and **ipecacuanha** was everyone's idea of a cold cure. Unfortunately people also bought the chlorodyne separately and used it as a cheap drink that gave the same effects as alcohol.

CHOKE DAMP. A name given by miners to the noxious gases filling the mines, especially after the use of explosives. See also **lead poisoning**. Coal miners in the West Midlands thought they could transfer the pain of their diseased lungs to the earth. A turf was dug out and the miner lay down taking deep breaths over the soil so the choke damp gases left the lungs for the earth.

See also **transference**.

CHOLERA. The cholera organism is found in the faeces of those suffering from the disease and infects others through contaminated **water** and food. The symptoms are severe watery **diarrhoea**, vomiting, cold and cramps leading to massive fluid loss and death within hours.

England in the 19th century was a breeding ground for this disease with poor hygiene, inadequate sanitation and contaminated water. For example, The Chelsea Water Company had its intake pipe in the Thames a few feet away from the outfall of a main London sewer. As *The Spectator* wrote, 'we are paying the companies

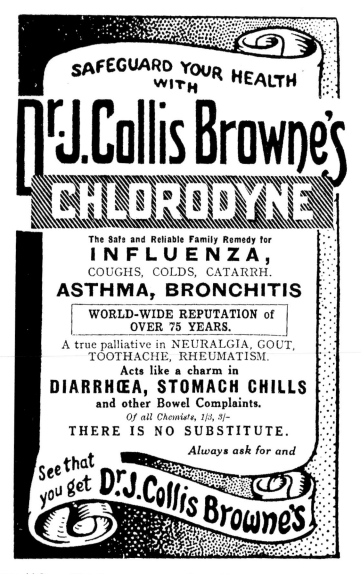

It was said Queen Victoria never went anywhere without a bottle of Dr J. Collis Browne's Chlorodyne. One of the most popular Victorian patent medicines and still going strong in the 1930s it contained chloroform, morphine and Indian hemp and could easily become addictive.

collectively £340,000 per annum for a more or less concentrated solution of native guano.'

Wave after wave of cholera hit England during the 1800s. It was first seen in Sunderland in October 1831 and moved south to London by January 1832. Again in 1848 cholera arrived via Newcastle, Liverpool and Carlisle and reached London where in 1849 some 14,000 people died. Further outbreaks meant that in London alone over 10,000 died in 1854 and over 5,000 in 1866.

There was no cure before the 20th century other than the complete overhaul of our sanitation and water supplies. The Public Health Act of 1848 began to address the problems of 'public nuisances' and clean piped water for all but legislation and any resulting action moved very slowly.

Remedies for cholera were based on getting the victim warmer so **ginger** and **cinnamon** made into a tea were drunk freely. The patient was also given hot water, enough to make them sick, and then a toasted oatcake soaked in a pint of boiling water and sipped. This last might have given some nourishment and replaced the liquid lost but really there was little to be done.

CINDER TEA. A red hot poker plunged into a cup of water made cinder tea for trapped **wind**. Before the advent of penicillin in the 1940s the remedy for a baby's chest infection was a cinder placed in a cup of water, cooled, then a drop of the cinder water given to the baby on a spoon. It was sometimes called sulphur water and when taken internally had some disinfectant properties but its most powerful action was as a laxative.

CINNAMON. The spice obtained from the bark of a species of laurel tree to be found in Asia. It has a stimulating effect on the stomach and acts as an antispasmodic which may explain its use in Victorian times for **cholera**. It was also thought to be beneficial in cases of **sea sickness** and trapped **wind**.

CLEAVERS. *Galium aparine*, otherwise known as goosegrass or Sticky Willie. Once used as a tea in the treatment of **measles**, supposedly to draw out the poisons of the infection. Still used today by herbalists because of its healing properties, especially for skin complaints.

CLOVES. Oil of cloves was applied to the gums for **toothache** or gumboils. All we knew then was that it worked by dulling the pain. Medical research tells us now the anaesthetic effect is attributed to the eugenol in the oil.

Sucking a clove was supposed to help anyone with an overfondness for drink as it helped to 'stay the craving'. Oil of cloves was generously rubbed into the chest for a **cold**.

CLYSTER. An old name for an **enema**. *The Family Physician* by Maximilian Hazlemore in 1794 gave the ingredients for a purging clyster as 6 ounces each of milk and water, 2 ounces each of fresh butter and brown sugar and 2 tablespoons of common **salt**. An extraordinary concoction!

COBWEB. Used since Roman times to cover **cuts** although it was not understood why it helped to heal so effectively. We now know that cobwebs contain a substance not unlike penicillin, and the proteins on the surface of the cobweb helps the blood to coagulate. A cobweb was always kept in the cellar for emergencies.

COFFEE. Drinking coffee was seen as almost as bad for you as **tea**. The Victorian Dr Browne wrote, 'Coffee possesses the narcotic principle, but in a lesser degree than tea; the same diseases follow its use.'

In the days when you died at home in your own bed the body was kept for a few days, laid out in an open coffin in the best parlour or front room, so that friends and relatives could visit to pay their last respects. To prevent any smell coming from the corpse, especially in hot weather, it was recommended to sprinkle fresh ground coffee in the room.

COLD BATHS. The unpleasantness of a cold bath might explain why it was thought such a good thing in effecting a cure and promoting an appetite. If you could think of no other way to treat the sick you could always fall back on a cold bath. Used in the treatment of conditions as diverse as blindness, **convulsions**, lung problems, **melancholy**, **rickets**, and the bite of a **mad dog**. For the latter you repeated the cold bath for 25 to 30 days successively. See also **tuberculosis**.

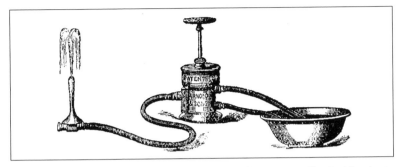

Arnold and Sons' 1876 Patent *Facilis Enema* in mahogany case, lined with velvet and priced at 25 shillings. You made up your own enema or clyster solution which went in the bowl and then sitting on the upright end you began to pump.
(By kind permission of the Thackray Museum, Leeds)

COLDS. We have all known the misery of a cold. These days we rely on pharmacists to help us out but in the past every household had a tried and tested way to prevent a cold or to relieve it once it had taken hold. Even today we are still searching for a cure for the common cold.

An old railwayman from Leeds who died in 1929 wrote in his account book, 'How to cure a cold in one night. Boil 1 ounce of **yarrow**, half an ounce of bruised **ginger** and 6 pennyworth of **cayenne** in 1 and a half pints of water until reduced down to half a pint. Take a wineglassful at bedtime. Spray 30 drops of eucalyptus oil in a pint of hot water and inhale for 10 minutes.'

Every unlikely commodity from the larder and kitchen cupboard was used to fight the cold. Country families cured their own bacon and a slice of fatty bacon was cut from the joint and made into a bacon **plaster**, attached to tapes and put on the chest. It was thought to keep the chest clear when you had a cold. Unfortunately if you wore it to school and it got warm the smell was awful.

A dash of **vinegar** was put in the bath if you felt a cold coming on.

If someone came to the house with a cold, you cut an **onion** in two and placed one half on a saucer in the living room and the other half on the window-ledge in the bedroom, leaving until shrivelled.

Drink **blackcurrant** tea or blackcurrant jam mixed with water to stop a cold from developing.

Castor oil and grated **nutmeg** was sprinkled onto brown paper. This was put onto the chest and pressed with a warm iron. You were then advised to wear your vest and liberty bodice over the top to keep it in place.

Swallow a mixture of **yeast**, sugar and butter.

To unblock a stuffed up nose, boiled **onions** were eaten to get the mucous membranes flowing.

Another remedy involved a teaspoon of **mustard** mixed into a paste with a little milk. Enough milk was then boiled to nearly fill a cup, the paste was added and the mixture stirred well. You proceeded straight to bed with this drink and a hot-water bottle.

A particularly disgusting cold cure involving **mustard**: sit with your feet in a mustard footbath whilst drinking black coffee with a spoonful of mustard mixed in it. To add to the feeling of misery sit over some hot water with a spoonful of mustard and breath in with a towel over your head.

An old Women's Institute book had a remedy requiring some skilful preparation, only to be expected of such an organisation. 'Take 4 ounces of whole **ginger**, 1 quart of water and the rind of a **lemon** and boil together for 1 hour, then strain. To each pint of this liquid add 12 ounces of sugar and juice of a **lemon**. Boil for 10 minutes; skim well, bottle and seal for future use. For a dose mix a small quantity with boiling water.'

The liquid from a **garlic** clove was rubbed onto the soles of the feet of a baby suffering from cold snuffles. An older child could have a mashed clove in a muslin bag tied round the neck.

Relief for a cold was to be had by drinking **raspberry** vinegar and the general rubbing in of such oils as **cloves, amber, a mixture of eucalyptus** and **camphor** and liberal amounts of **goose grease** and **camphor**. See also **balsam, daisy** and **mutton suet**.

The old saying, 'Ne'er cast a clout till May be out,' is followed by the second less well known line supplied to me by Mrs Barbara

Arm of Leicestershire: 'Or you'll catch a cold in June.'

If unlucky enough to catch a cold after this sound advice, Mrs Arm supplied me with the following cold cure. Drink a cup of hot milk with whisky, a spoonful of **honey** and some shredded suet mixed in. Pity about the suet!

COLLIS BROWNE. See **chlorodyne**.

COLTSFOOT. *Tussilago farfara*. The name Tussilago is from the Latin word *tussis* – cough. The Romans burned the leaves and roots and swallowed the smoke. Cornish miners smoked it as a herbal tobacco to prevent lung disease. It is an astringent, expectorant herb that relaxes spasms and controls coughing. It also reduces inflammation and soothes irritated tissues and has been used for deep **cuts, eczema** and **rheumatic** joints.

See also **pestilent wort**.

COMFREY. *Symphytum officinale*. Also known as knitbone, knitback, bruisewort and ass ear. Nicholas Culpepper wrote in 1653 that it was 'special good for ruptures and broken bones'. He also made the unlikely claim that if comfrey was boiled together with pieces of flesh in a pan it would join the flesh together again!

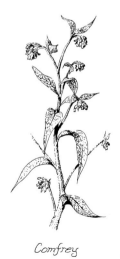

Comfrey

It is undoubtedly a powerful and useful herb. The leaf contains allentoin, a protein encouraging cell division, which is responsible for its healing properties. A **poultice** was the favourite way of using comfrey. The leaves were boiled for a short time and then made into a poultice, placed on the swelling and held there by a bandage.

Comfrey leaves were once eaten as a vegetable and regularly made into an **infusion** and drunk as a tea. Medical research into this herb has now found that the alkaloids in comfrey can cause liver damage when taken internally. Comfrey tea was drunk to treat any **kidney complaint** and is an example of how some of the old remedies were probably quite harmful!

COMMONPLACE BOOK. A small intimate book kept in the past by women in which to record remedies, good recipes, household hints, perhaps a favourite poem, wise sayings or a prayer. Men to a lesser extent kept these little books but they were far more likely to have mainly household accounts written up, or if in farming, remedies for the animals. I have been very privileged to read many of these books for my research and they are greatly cherished by the family members who now hold them.

COMPLAINTS OF ANY SORT. The optimism in this recommendation from a 1930s home remedy book is quite touching. '**Vinegar** mixed with **honey** with a pinch of **mustard** in it, and taken freely, stops any complaint from advancing. For any complaint a mixture of breadcrumbs, mustard and vinegar is good to use inwardly.' This must come into the category of: if you believed it was doing you some good, it just might.

COMPLEXION. *The Lady's World* of 1898 placed great emphasis on a healthy complexion. 'Many a girl, with quite plain looking features, is rendered brilliant and attractive by her beautiful complexion. On the other hand, there are numbers of women, having excellently chiselled features, who yet fail to please the eye, simply because they are the unfortunate owner of a sallow, muddy complexion.' Howard Green MRCS who wrote this failed to mention the condition of his own complexion.

An old Northamptonshire rhyme gave some straightforward advice:

Enos Fruit Salts

4 ozs Carbonate of Soda
2 ozs Tartaric acid
2 do Epson Salts
2 " Cream of Tartar
2 " Bi Carbonate of Potash
4 " Powdered Sugar

To be well Powdered, and
The Salts & Potash to be
well dried before Mixing,
Bottle airtight,
Dose one Teaspoonfull in
a ½ Glass of Cold Water.

A very good Receipt for Health

A page from the leather-bound commonplace book belonging to a farmer, Mr Edward Brown, dated 1895. There were cures in the front for humans and even more cures in the back for his animals.

'With spinach and leek,
Lily cheeks in a week.'

A remedy still in use by several elderly ladies I know – drink hot **cabbage** water.

Many people have remarked to me on the beautiful skin of their grandmothers, even in old age. These ladies had one thing in common; they all used only carbolic soap and washed in cold rainwater, often having to break the ice in the morning. Lessons could be learned from these simple ways. See also **parsley** and **wild strawberry**.

CONCEPTION. Right up to the Second World War it was thought by lying on your right side during intercourse you would conceive a boy and on your left a girl.

On the East Coast having intercourse when the tide was coming in would ensure conception. See also **contraception** for the reverse.

It was believed the mother's 'system' could be manipulated into having the sex of the child you wanted. You needed an acid 'system' for a girl, therefore you douched with a solution of boracic acid and an alkaline one for a boy so you applied a solution of **bicarbonate of soda**.

A red haired baby meant you had made love during the mother's monthly period!

CONSTIPATION. Costiveness or constipation was an obsession in the past and the state of one's **bowels** was a daily consideration and worry. **Aperients**, **enemas** and **purgatives** were liberally and frequently administered, and not just by the medical profession, in the event that there was little else to be done in the case of most illnesses. Middle class meals laden with meat and puddings and little in the way of fruit and vegetables meant a sluggish system: roughage was an unknown word. The evil of constipation was seen as the root cause of bad health. See also **aloes, Beecham's pills** and **water**.

CONSUMPTION. A word used by ordinary people for the illness **tuberculosis**. From the Latin *consumptio* meaning 'a wasting', describing the physical wasting away of the body.

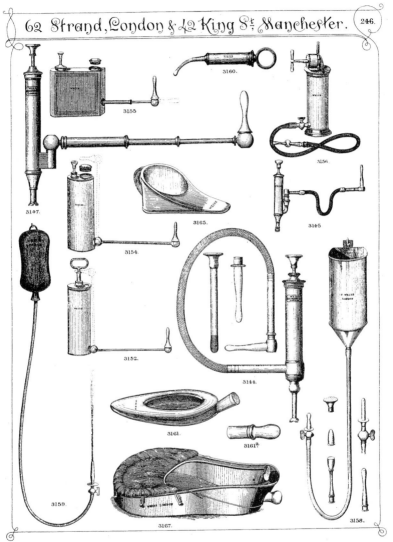

62 Strand, London & 42 King St, Manchester. 246.

3160.
3155
3156.
3147.
3165.
3145
3154.
3152.
3144.
3161.
3161ᵃ
3159.
3167.
3158.

A 1889 catalogue reflecting the Victorians' obsession with constipation and their bowels. These enemas, syringes and douches were all available to the public and were thought to be indispensable items for home use by the middle classes. Number 3155 was disguised as a book for a gentleman to keep in his library ready for use. Number 3156 gave enormous pressure which would have done untold damage. (By kind permission of the Thackray Museum, Leeds)

CONTRACEPTION. A very hit and miss affair with women passing on what had worked for them. The middle classes in Victorian England practised coitus interruptus but many working class men thought this to be most unnatural.

The most commonly held myth was that you could not get pregnant 'the first time'. Many young girls found to their cost that this was not the case.

If you lived by the sea, you could make sure you only had intercourse when the tide was going out.

Jumping, sneezing and exercising after intercourse would prevent conception.

Inserting one's wedding ring into the uterus was the precursor of the intra-uterine device.

Other household items once inserted to prevent a pregnancy included cheese and a rag soaked in **vinegar**.

CONVULSIONS. Known as febrile convulsions in children, sometimes occurring with a high temperature. The correct treatment is to remove the child's clothes and keep him cool.

Treatment in the past must have been alarming for the child. According to archive material collected by the Northampton Living Memory Group, 'Place the child at once in a hot **mustard** bath and wrap a cold wet cloth around his head. Get him dry, then roll him in a blanket and put him to bed. Comfort him gently and give an **enema** of soap suds. Should this prove difficult a dose of **castor oil** will produce the desired effect.' See also **cold baths**.

CORNS. Corns are mostly caused by badly fitting shoes. In large, poor families shoes were meant to last and were passed down from child to child. This was the worst possible thing for feet as no one had a shoe that fitted them properly. Corns were treated with a variety of homemade potions:

Cover the corn with **lemon** juice mixed with **Epsom salts**.

Mix flour and **mustard** powder into a paste with a little cold water and then add 1 pint of hot water and soak your feet in this once a week.

Rub the corn with a little oil of **peppermint**, the side of a matchbox or **turpentine**.

Crush an **ivy** leaf and place onto the corn, covering it with an elastoplast. Leave for two weeks and do not get it wet.

Fasten a hot roast **garlic** to the corn.

For a homemade corn plaster fold some brown paper into a thickness of four pieces and make an incision. Insert the corn into it and apply a piece of boiled salted **carrot**.

A popular patent remedy was Black Jack which came in small tins with the Union Jack on the lid.

From Wiltshire came the advice to boil a potato in its skin, eat the potato but leave the skin which is then bound onto the corn for 12 hours.

In Cornwall they preferred an altogether harsher way of dealing with their corns – beating them regularly with a branch of holly.

COUGH MEDICINES. Industrial pollution, bad housing, poor general health, city smogs and the cigarette meant that few people were without a cough. **Camphorated oil** and **goose grease** were rubbed directly onto the chest or applied to brown paper which was then placed next to the chest and held in place by a vest or liberty bodice. Other items placed on the chest might be a **mustard plaster**, a rabbit skin, a piece of blanket preferably red in colour, or a **poultice** of tallow fat and **nutmeg**.

The medical profession became increasingly alarmed with cough mixtures containing **laudanum** and **paregoric,** the great favourites of the Victorians. Even cough mixtures for children, such as in an old recipe book produced by a Presbyterian church in Northumberland, contained paregoric. At least if you made them at home you knew what went into them, or thought you did, and they were significantly cheaper. Homemade cough remedies were made up in the kitchen and every family had a cure they would 'swear by'.

Until very recently a popular cure involving **turnips** was still being made. You took a washed turnip, cut it into slices and placed them in a large basin layered with brown sugar. You then covered the whole thing and put it in a warm oven for several hours. The sugar melted and from the turnip oozed a juice and the mixture made an excellent cough medicine. It tasted delicious but smelled awful.

Or you could substitute an **onion** for the turnip.

John Wesley in his *Primitive Physic* too was a believer in the turnip but he also much favoured cold water: 'Use the cold bath – It seldom fails.'

Many ingredients of homemade cough medicine had a soothing, lubricant effect and the alcohol content was a relaxant. Some had so much alcohol in them that after a few doses you would have known little pain.

From Barnsley comes a good cough medicine dispensed from a little shop in the front room of a house in the 1890s. Mix 3 eggs, 4 ounces of **honey**, half a pint of port wine and 3 tablespoons of rum.

Another pleasant cough medicine needing alcohol. Three tablespoons each of whisky and **honey**, 2 dessertspoons of glycerine, the juice of a **lemon**, shake all together and take a dessertspoon when needed.

For cough syrup mix 1 tablespoon each of **castor oil**, **vinegar**, and Golden Syrup and take half a teaspoon. Other variations added butter and brown sugar or melted bought sweets like mint rock.

A cough medicine needing a significant amount of courage to take was a teaspoon of Golden Syrup and 2 teaspoons of grated suet in a cup of warm milk. Considered to be especially good for a wheezing child having difficulty breathing.

A cough medicine from the 1920s made from ingredients bought from the chemist: 2 pennyworth each of **liquorice**, oil of almonds, **peppermint**, aniseed and **paregoric**, some white wine **vinegar** and 1lb of treacle. Dissolve the liquorice in a pint of boiling water, add the treacle and stir well. When cool add all the other ingredients and bottle. To give an extra 'kick' **cayenne** and **ipecacuanha** were added.

A nastier cough medicine was made from boiling liquorice sticks slowly with **linseed** oil.

Other lubricants were oil of almonds, syrup of violets with **squills** and **rose hip** syrup.

For working people living in towns the use of herbs for treating a cough were strictly limited. A sugar lump with 2 drops of **turpentine** was an easy remedy.

In the country you were made to walk through a flock of sheep to clear a cough or you might have used a very limited range of herbs such as **coltsfoot** tea sweetened with a spoonful of honey, **dandelion** or **ground ivy**.

CRAMP. Painful night cramps were claimed to be cured by sleeping with a dozen corks and for good measure you carried them around with you!

In 19th century Shropshire and in the more remote areas of the North, to prevent night cramp, on going to bed you left your shoes in the shape of a T. This was known as a Tau cross from the cross shape of the Greek letter *tau*.

CROUP. Literally means 'to croak' and describes the hoarse, noisy breathing and coughing in a small child. The traditional method of dealing with this distressing illness was to put the child into a hot bath in which some **mustard** had been dissolved and cover the bath with a tent made from a blanket. The child would inhale the steam while sitting in the bath – an altogether scary experience. Even more unpleasant was a teaspoon of **goose grease** three times a day.

CULPEPPER. Nicholas Culpepper (1616–1654), the English medical writer and astrologer. In 1640 he set up in London as a physician and astrologer – the two seen by many as dependent on each other. In 1652 he wrote a herbal *The English Physitian* describing the medicinal action of over 300 herbs – as he saw it. Unfortunately he also combined this wisdom with astrology and the **Doctrine of Signatures**.

CUPPING. A method of **blood-letting** causing dilation of the superficial blood vessels. Small cups were heated and placed on the skin, usually on the back. As they cooled the skin became swollen and drawn into the vacuum and when the cups were removed the skin was pricked to draw blood.

CUTS. A traditional cure for a deep cut was a **cobweb** placed directly onto the cut. A cobweb was always left in the cellar or the workshop in case of accidents.

An old farming remedy left 2 thick slices of bread on the dairy floor until a mould appeared. The mouldy bread was made into a paste and placed on the cut. There was something similar in the Black Country where a cut was wrapped with the mould from the top of homemade jam.

It must have been a brave person who first tried out these early forms of **penicillin**.

Brown paper soaked in **vinegar** and bound onto the cut (as in Jack and Jill).

A puff-ball fungus placed over the cut was said to heal without leaving a scar. See also **coltsfoot**.

A cloth with **soap** and sugar on it, left on the cut for 24 hours.

In the First World War wounded men, miles from anywhere, placed moss onto a deep cut.

A dab of **turpentine** or **honey** healed a cut.

A more repugnant old cure from the West Midlands had small children rubbing 'snot' onto a cut. See also **saliva**.

Fishermen bound their cuts with yarn impregnated with **tar**.

A cigarette paper was placed over a small cut caused by using a cut throat razor when shaving.

CYSTITIS. John Wesley in his *Primitive Physic* described it accurately as: '**urine** by drops with heat and pain.' He advised quite sensibly drinking only lemonade but his use of **apples** seems strange to us now. 'Beat up the pulp of 5 or 6 roasted apples with near a quart of water. Take it lying down. It commonly cures before morning.' See also **barley water** and **wood betony**.

D

First the Distiller, then the Doctor, then the Undertaker.

DAISY. *Bellis perennis*. The common daisy – overlooked, scorned and in our lawns treated with weedkiller. The daisy has been used for centuries in medicines for its healing and expectorant properties. **Gerard** in his 1597 *Herball* recommended applying daisies mixed with butter to painful joints.

In the 1880s in Wiltshire the field daisy was widely used in an **infusion** for a **cold**.

DANDELION. *Taraxacum officinale*. A powerful diuretic plant; the French call it '*pissenlit*', wet-the-bed. The leaves and roots flavour soft drinks like dandelion and **burdock**; the roots dried, roasted and ground make a caffeine-free coffee substitute; the juice from the stalk is effective in getting rid of **warts** and **verrucas** and the flowers can be made into wine.

Dandelion tea was considered to be a tonic and good for **indigestion**. A recipe from the 1920s advised: 'Take the roots of 6 dandelions, having first cut off the leaves, wash and scrape the roots, cut them into short pieces, pour over a pint of boiling water, let it stand for 12 hours, then strain through muslin and dose a wineglassful a day.'

A **cough** remedy from the 1880s recommended 1 pennyworth each of dandelion and **ground ivy** to be boiled in 3 pints of water down to 1 pint. Drink a wineglass 3 times a day.

To think of the money and effort spent on clearing our lawns of these so called weeds – throw away the weed killer and allow them to flourish!

DANDRUFF. This expensive cure for dandruff was used in the early 1900s but only by the well-heeled – the poor had more to worry about than dandruff. Mix 1 pint each of bay rum and soft water and 1 teaspoon of salt, shake before using each night. The poor might have used a solution of **borax**.

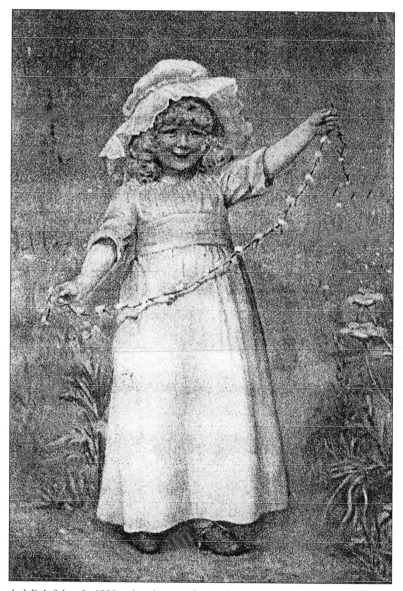

A delightful early 1900s advertisement for the famous and very effective Daisy Powders which treated headaches and contained the analgesic acetanilide, a white crystalline powder. (By kind permission of the Thackray Museum, Leeds)

DEAFNESS. It was believed that possible causes of deafness were blowing your nose too hard or sitting with your back to the window.

Wax in the ear was dealt with effectively by alcohol dropped in and loosening the hard wax. A mixture of oil of **cloves**, the juice from the **foxglove** and rum dropped onto some cotton wool and left in the ear did little harm and might even have helped.

Other items people placed happily in their ears to cure deafness were less effective: the juice from **ground ivy**, a clove of **garlic** dipped in **honey**, warm **sage** tea, **salt** water, **onion** juice and crushed wild **mint**.

DECOCTION. A method of extracting the essence of a plant by boiling. Used for the tougher part of the herb such as the root or stem. Add 1 ounce (25g) of chopped herb to 1 pint (600ml) of boiling water, simmer for 30 minutes. Strain, cool and drink the same day.

DELICATE PEOPLE. It was a common problem in large Victorian middle class families for at least one member to be a little 'delicate'. Mostly it was a female but sometimes a male, especially an only son of a dominant mother. Those labelled as 'delicate' were not expected to work or marry but had the luxury of a family who could keep them.

The women stayed at home, often as company for elderly parents. Much of their trouble stemmed from tight corsets and bad drains. Early water closets installed in the homes of the better off failed to have adequate drainage and a cocktail of foul sewer gas and bacteria was pulled into the house by the draught from open fires. Women and servants who spent more time in the house were liable to non-specific **headaches**, **sore throats** and depressed health. The image of the Victorian lady lying prostrate on her chaise longue was a very real one.

General advice for the 'delicate' was to take light suppers and drink plenty of **water**, not always good advice as most water supplies in towns were highly polluted with effluent. When this failed to work a short stay in one of the many **spa** towns might make you feel better, only for a relapse on returning to the old unsanitary conditions.

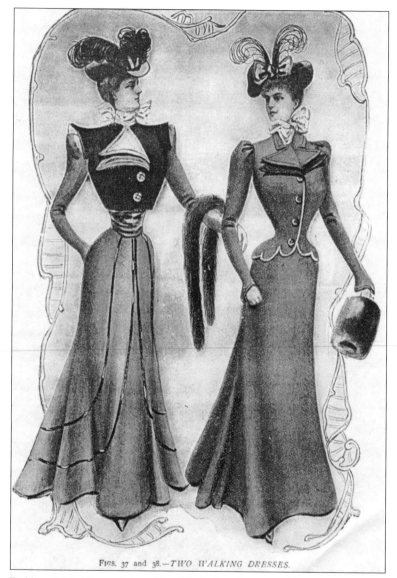

FIGS. 37 and 38.—*TWO WALKING DRESSES.*

Fashion dictated tiny waists and the tight lacing of corsets. This in turn meant internal problems like indigestion, liver and bowel problems, palpitations and fainting. These walking dresses from *The Lady's World* of 1899 may be exaggerated but it was the look every fashionable woman wanted.

DEPRESSION. It was widely believed that depression was caused by **indigestion**.

The Family Physician of 1794 was most specific as to the causes: 'Intense thinking, violent passions or affections of the mind as love, fear, joy, grief.' The writer advised: 'The diet should consist chiefly of vegetables of a cooling and opening quality. Animal food especially salted or smoked dried fish or flesh ought to be avoided. The most proper drink is water, whey or small beer. **Tea** and **coffee** are improper.'

DERBYSHIRE NECK. See **goitre**.

DIABETES. A condition in which the body cannot properly use sugar and carbohydrates because the pancreas is not producing enough insulin. Before this was fully understood the medical profession believed drinking too much inferior **tea** caused diabetes. See also **pennyroyal** and **pisse prophet**.

DIARRHOEA. The delicate balance of their **bowels** occupied the English to an extent unimaginable these days. Half the country were taking **aperients** and **purgatives**, the other half suffering from an excess were trying to 'stop themselves up'. Serious diarrhoea was a symptom of the dreaded **cholera** and **typhoid fever**.

Taking flour and water was an old army trick to stop diarrhoea.

Drink tea made from **raspberry** leaf, **chamomile** or **wood betony**.

A very old remedy discovered in the Thackray Medical Museum in Leeds advised sitting on a chamber pot containing **chamomile** flowers boiled in milk.

If the diarrhoea was caused by an irritant or indigestible substance a dose of **castor oil** was given.

DIETING. In the past we were not so obsessed with the cult of thinness. The working poor were more interested in getting enough to eat and being overweight was not a problem for them. However fashionable Victorian women wanted a curvaceous figure, with a tiny waist and full bosom. To achieve this women willingly had themselves fastened into life threatening corsets or 'stays', the ferocity of the tightness leaving them gasping for breath, barely able to bend. The consequences in health terms are not hard to imagine; internal organs squashed, lungs punctured, ribs deformed and incontinence. But to gain some respite and leave your corsets off in public was thought vulgar and labelled you as not 'nice'.

A Victorian undertaker called William Banting devised a high-protein, low-carbohydrate diet which together with the awful corset was highly effective. Following his regime was known as 'banting'.

It was a popular myth that eating radish, **garlic** and spices or anything causing internal heat and perspiration would help you lose weight.

Sensible advice on the subject of dieting:

> If you wish to grow thinner, diminish your dinner,
> And take to light claret instead of pale ale;
> Look down with an utter contempt upon butter,
> And never touch bread till it's toasted – or stale.
> (Henry Leigh from *A Day of Wishing*, 1869)

DIPHTHERIA. A major killer of young people until the launch of an immunisation campaign in 1940 which virtually eliminated the disease. Starting with a **sore throat** and **fever**, a membrane grew across the throat making breathing difficult. Toxins lead to heart failure and paralysis of the muscles for breathing and swallowing.

It was a constant worry whenever there was an epidemic. Every sore throat was treated with suspicion and the child was rushed off to the local isolation hospital. Diphtheria epidemics were most common in autumn and winter and mainly affected school children. On arriving home from school, a preventative measure was to stand over a fire shovel of red hot coals, sprinkled with yellow **sulphur** powder, breathing in the fumes. The sulphur acted as a **disinfectant**. Drinking **olive oil** was thought to help keep the throat clear.

If none of these worked and the child caught diphtheria then further disinfectant fumes were made at home by heating a tin mug containing **tar** and **turpentine**.

DISINFECTANT. **Tar** from the side of the road was a readily available disinfectant but fresh ground **coffee** was thought even better. Flowers of **sulphur** was also used, either blown down the throat or sprinkled on the fire.

DIZZINESS. A symptom for any number of illnesses but a 1930s home remedy book advised drinking **sage** tea.

DOCK LEAF. A well known cure for **nettle rash** but chewing it first made the dock leaf more effective. The alkaline secretions of the smaller 'sour dockings', especially when added to some **saliva,** can be very soothing. For good measure while you were doing all this you said the old rhyme:

> 'Nettle out, dock in,
> Dock remove nettle sting.
> In dock, out nettle,
> Don't let the blood settle.'

A clump of dock leaves was always grown in the country cottage garden as a substitute for lavatory paper when the newspaper squares had run out in the old outdoor privy.

See also **legs**.

DOCTRINE OF SIGNATURES. For centuries medicine was based on the belief that the colour and shape of a herb was God's way of indicating what healing properties that herb might have. Famous examples are the lesser celandine (**pilewort**); *pulmonaria* (lungwort) – its spotted leaves look like a diseased lung; *Hepatica noblis* (liverwort) – its leaves resemble a liver; *Euphrasia officinalis* (eyebright) the flower has the colouring of a bloodshot eye.

DOG BITE. See **mad dog bite**.

DONKEY. Often thought of as stupid and obstinate the donkey holds a peculiar place in medical myth. The cross on a donkey's back was thought to be a holy marking as Jesus chose this humble animal to enter Jerusalem on Palm Sunday. This may explain the widespread belief that to pass a child under the belly of a donkey, preferably 9 times, would bring a cure for **whooping cough**. Even hairs taken from the donkey's back and sewn into a bag worn round the neck were considered potent enough for a cure.

Donkey owners at seaside towns continued to earn money in the winter by taking poorly children for a ride. It was the belief in the donkey rather than the sea air that led mothers and their children to the beach in winter.

DOUCHE. A stream of water directed onto the body or into a body cavity for cleansing or medical purposes. The word also referred to the instrument by which you administered the douche. For Victorian ladies with access to some form of a bathroom the douche was used to prevent pregnancy immediately after sexual intercourse.

From the middle of the 1800s onwards the Douche Bath was increasingly popular with water forcefully applied to those taking a 'Water Cure' in a variety of inventive ways. A powerful icy jet of water was directed at the painful part and to this end a water tank was constructed some 20 feet above the patient to obtain a decent head of pressure. Sometimes it was so powerful that a strong hat was worn to protect the head!

DOVER POWDER. A mixture of **ipecacuanha** and **opium** which was very popular as a sedative for feverish **coughs** and **colds**. Not surprisingly with those ingredients it could become addictive. The powder was named after the man who first prepared it, Captain Thomas Dover (1660–1742). He was an interesting character, a privateer who was part of the expedition that rescued Alexander Selkirk from an island off the coast of Chile and whose story became Daniel Defoe's *Robinson Crusoe*.

DRAUGHTS. Sitting in a cold draught is rather unpleasant and unnecessary now in our centrally heated homes and offices. Once sitting in a draught was regarded as the height of folly. *The Lady's World* in 1898 explained: 'It is a frequent excitant of disease for the blood gets chilled and a cold is caught.' In the better class of house you always sat with your feet on a footstool to escape the draughts round the feet as the coal fire sucked in the cold air under the door.

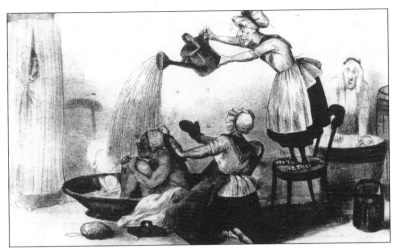

The ever popular douche where a stream of water is directed at the body for cleansing or medical purposes. Just one of the many and varied health treatments available at spa towns. This cartoon from a humorous Victorian booklet *The Sure Water Cure* pokes fun at 'The Ladies Sitting Douche'. (By kind permission of Harrogate Museums and Art Gallery Service)

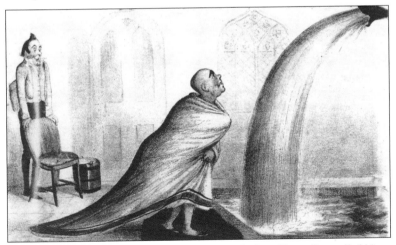

A cartoon from the humorous Victorian booklet, *The Sure Water Cure* called 'A Deuced Douche.' The writer suggested if it was the force of water that cured why not construct a douche under Niagara Falls but the 'Water Doctors' should try it first as 'Drowning would be a natural death for them!' (By kind permission of Harrogate Museums and Art Gallery Service)

DROPSY. The word 'dropsy' was given as the cause of death on many old death certificates but in fact this is not a disease. It is when an abnormal amount of fluid accumulates beneath the skin, known now as oedema, and it can be due to several illnesses. The most common would be heart disease, due to the inadequate pumping action of the heart and Bright's disease where the kidneys are failing in their function.

For centuries Shropshire folklore knew of the benefits of the **foxglove** in treating dropsy and the leaf was used in the form of a tea. However, as all parts of the foxglove are extremely poisonous it must have been a perilous remedy to use.

Dropsy was a common symptom and John Wesley in his *Primitive Physic* accurately described it and gave many remedies, none of which would have helped. Some would have been downright dangerous. 'Apply green **dock leaves** to the joints and soles of the feet, changing them once a day. Abstain from all drink for 30 days. To ease your thirst hold often on your tongue, a thin small slice of toasted bread dipt in Brandy, or wash the mouth with juice of lemons.'

His advice to drink half a pint of **sea water** every morning and evening must have added much misery to the already sick.

DYSENTERY. An older name for this distressing infection of the **bowels** was the 'bloody flux', an apt description of the watery stools streaked with blood. **Diarrhoea**, violent griping pains, vomiting and **wind** led to extreme weakness and even death. Dysentery was rife in unsanitary, overcrowded slums and gaols. Soldiers fighting in the past often succumbed and many a battle has been lost to dysentery rather than a superior foe.

There was little to be done on the battlefield but at home an egg beaten lightly with sugar and swallowed in one go was thought to calm the digestive system. See also **benjamin** and **primrose**.

DYSPEPSIA. Another word for **indigestion** or upset stomach.

E

Exercise is indispensably necessary to health and long life.

EARACHE. Old remedies relied on applying warmth to the painful ear or cheek and a variety of foodstuffs were placed in or against the ear, all capable of holding the heat.

A small lump of hot potato or the middle of a warm **onion** was inserted into the ear.

Warm **olive oil** was dripped from a knitting needle into the ear or onto cotton wool which was then inserted. The oil was also rubbed onto the back of the ear. A warm scarf wrapped round the head kept the heat in.

A drop of warm whisky dropped from a spoon made a crackling noise in the ear as it dissolved the wax.

Hot toasted bread was placed against the ear or a **poultice** of baked **apple**.

A heap of salt on a shovel was heated over the fire and when hot put in a sock and held against the ear.

The ear was rubbed with a dry flannel or bathed with a warm **decoction** of **chamomile** flowers and **poppy** heads.

For earache brought on by the cold John Wesley in his *Primitive Physic* advised: 'Boil **rue**, or **rosemary**, or **garlick** [sic] and let the steam go into the ear thro' a funnel,' and for ringing noises in the ear he suggested dropping in some juice from an **onion** or filling the ear with bruised **hyssop**.

One can only wonder at the circumstances in which you would need the following advice. It was given to me by a Yorkshirewoman whose mother took a job as a lady's maid at the Grand Hotel, Scarborough in the 1890s. Being resourceful, she noted down in her **commonplace book** everything she had found useful in the course of her work. 'If gnats or earwigs get into the ear, a puff of tobacco smoke will render them helpless and afterwards the ear can be washed out with a little warm water.'

The Family Physician of 1794 recommended a dose of **nitre** and **rhubarb** as a **purgative** in the mistaken belief that attending to the **bowels** would cure earache.

EASTER-LEDGE PUDDING. Sometimes known as Herb Pudding or Nettle and Passion Dock Pudding. A springtime speciality for Northern mothers who served it to their families as a medicinal treat. It acted as a mild **purgative** but also pepped up a sluggish system after a long cold winter. The principal ingredient was bistort leaves, a plant containing tannin with astringent properties. Other names for bistort were Passion Dock or Easterman Giant, a corruption of Easter-mangient, meaning a plant to be eaten at Easter. Sometimes young **nettle** leaves were added to the bistort.

I am assured by those who have eaten it that this pudding is quite delicious.

Easter-Ledge Pudding

Around Eastertime pick young nettle tops and bistort leaves. Wash and cut up and fry in butter with a handful of oatmeal. (I am told that at this stage it resembles a cowpat.) In parts of Cumbria **dandelion** leaves were added for good measure. Add a couple of eggs and eat with fried bacon.

Guaranteed to put a spring into anyone's step!

ECZEMA. A **poultice** of **burdock** leaves or the juice from fresh **watercress** on the inflamed skin was said to soothe.

To cure this distressing skin complaint Berkshire gypsies advised bathing in **sea water**. Dartmoor gypsies thought milk or cream from a red cow would effect relief but it was not made clear whether you should wash in it or drink it. Unwise for the lactose intolerant! See also **coltsfoot, ground ivy** and **wells**.

ELDER. A tree associated with magic, medicine and folklore since ancient times which explains its use in curing **warts**. An elder tree was often planted next to an outdoor privy to keep away the flies and it was believed unlucky to cut one down. All parts of the elder have been used in the past with probably mixed success.

The leaves and raw berries are harmful if eaten but **Gerard** recommended in his *Herball* that the seeds be taken in a drop of wine as a cure for **dropsy** and also to lose weight. As the seeds or raw berries would probably make you sick perhaps that is what he meant by weight loss.

ELDERBERRY. The fruits are used as flavouring or made into a cordial and contain large amounts of vitamin C when fresh. Elderberry juice mixed with port wine was said to banish the pain of **sciatica** and **neuralgia**. Homemade elderberry cordial was always on hand in country kitchens for anyone suffering with a **cold**, **influenza** or a **fever**. Elderberries contain viburnic acid which induces perspiration and was thought useful in cases of **bronchitis**. Elderberry wine was once so popular as a medicine that whole orchards were planted in Kent and the berries sold for winemaking.

Margaret Hopper's Elderberry Cordial

Gather ripe berries on a dry day, remove the stalks and put the berries into jars. Stand the jars in boiling water until the juice runs. Strain off the juice and to every quart add 1 ounce of bruised whole **ginger**, 1 teaspoon of **cloves** and 2 pounds of sugar. Simmer gently for 1 hour, leave until cold then strain through muslin and bottle.

ELDERFLOWER. The flower heads of the **elder** tree contain anti-inflammatory properties. They can be fried in batter, used to flavour jellies and jam and made into elderflower 'champagne'.

Elderflower Champagne

Pick 2 heads of elderflower when in full bloom and put into a bowl with the juice and rind of a lemon (make sure there is no white pith left on the rind), 24 ounces of sugar and 2 tablespoons of white wine vinegar. Pour on 8 pints of cold water and leave for 24 hours. Strain into bottles, cork firmly and lay them on their sides and after 2 weeks it should be sparkling and ready to drink.

ELECTUARY. A soft paste of any unpalatable medicine mixed with **honey** or syrup to be taken internally. See also **piles**.

EMBROCATION. See also **liniment**. A mixture for external use for **muscular aches**, **rheumatism** or **sprains** which usually gave relief, partly because of the rubbing action, but also the ingredients had a counter-irritant effect, that is replacing a nasty pain with a nice pain.

Grandmother's Embrocation

Place half a pint of **turpentine** and 1 egg into a large bottle. Cork it and shake until it becomes cream. Gradually add 1 pint of vinegar and a small tablespoonful of liquid ammonia and bottle for use. Other remedies substituted 30 drops of **camphor** for the ammonia.

ENEMA. See **clyster**.

EPILEPSY. Also known as the 'falling sickness' or the 'sacred disease'. This illness has been recognised since ancient times and had about it an aura of mystery. Family doctors in the past would firmly advise the person not to marry. Sadly all too often people suffering from epilepsy were sent to an asylum.

The Royal Family displayed the attitude of the times when Prince John, the last child, born in 1905, to the future King George V and Queen Mary, developed epilepsy. He spent his short life kept out of sight on the Sandringham estate until he died in 1919.

The condition was not understood and families were secretive and ashamed of any member who suffered. I know of one grandmother, who on learning her granddaughter had developed epilepsy, declared, 'Well she didn't get it from our side of the family.'

John Wesley in his *Primitive Physic* described the condition and had several remedies: 'In the falling sickness the patient falls to the ground, either quite stiff, or convulsed all over, utterly senseless gnashing his teeth, and foaming at the mouth. Use the cold bath for a month daily. Or take a teaspoonful of **Peony** Root dried and grated fine, morning and evening for 3 months.'

Other recommendations were **laudanum**, **nutmeg**, a diet consisting entirely of milk, blowing powdered **ginger** up the nose during the fit and dried earthworms. Finally Wesley entered the realms of superstition: 'If **mistletoe** is gathered on the first day of the new moon without being touched by iron or allowed to fall on the ground, it is said to be a certain cure for falling sickness. Make the wood and leaves into a **decoction**.' This last must have been extremely dangerous as the mistletoe is highly toxic if eaten.

Wearing mistletoe was believed to be a cure for epilepsy and protection against witchcraft and possession by the Devil. The link between the two in the medieval mind was an easy one to make and prayers for a cure were made to the Saints Valentine, Sebastian and Vitus. Even up to the 1930s an ounce each of mistletoe and **valerian** root together with **horehound** was still seen as helpful in epilepsy.

I have found an unusual 19th century cure in several areas of the country skilfully combining superstition and religion. In parts of the West Country, Shropshire, the Forest of Dean and Yorkshire the person with epilepsy sat in the church porch during the Sunday service and 30 married men handed over a penny each on leaving the church. This money was then exchanged for half a crown (2/6d) which was melted down and made into a ring for the epileptic to wear. Some Church of England clergymen, quite naturally, were unhappy with the superstitious use of the church porch.

EPSOM SALTS. Sulphate of magnesia obtained originally from a mineral spring at Epsom and used extensively since the mid 1600s for disorders of the stomach and **bowels**. See also **boils**.

ERYNGIUM MARITIMUM. Otherwise known as sea holly. From early times this plant was thought to have healing properties especially when used against the **King's evil**, **ague** and serpent bites. Colchester was famous for harvesting the root which in the 17th and 18th centuries was conserved in sugar and eaten as a lozenge with supposedly aphrodisiac properties. Falstaff in Shakespeare's *The Merry Wives of Windsor* asked for the sky to rain 'eringoes' and 'kissing comfits'.

ERYSIPELAS. A highly contagious streptococcal skin infection known in the Middle Ages as The Rose or St Anthony's Fire on account of the heat and redness of the skin. It could be fatal before the advent of **penicillin** and spread like wildfire in unsanitary places like gaols, army camps – and hospitals.

John Wesley in his *Primitive Physic* advised drinking **tar** water or a pint of **sea water** every morning.

A home remedy book from the 1930s recommended adding 2 sprigs of **wormwood** and ¼ ounce each of **senna** and **chamomile** flowers to a pint of boiling water and drinking the result freely.

EUCALYPTUS OIL. A volatile oil from the many kinds of gum tree to be found in Australia. Eucalyptus oils were produced commercially in Australia from 1860 by Yorkshireman Joseph Bosisto, an immigrant. Eucalyptus oil was marketed as a **cold** cure and a good decongestant but it is now recognised as toxic. However, in the past that did not stop our families from rubbing generous amounts onto their chests.

EUPHORBIA. *Euphorbia hirta* also known as spurge. This garden plant was once a well known cure for a **wart**. The juice from the stem is a strong irritant and when rubbed onto the wart caused blisters which replaced the wart.

EYAM. The Great Plague of 1665 decimated the once remote village of Eyam in Derbyshire. The fleas carrying the **bubonic plague** arrived in a box of clothes and within months 260 of the village were dead. The young rector of Eyam, William Mompesson, persuaded the remaining villagers to stay in a self imposed quarantine in order not to spread the plague to the nearby towns of Derby and Chesterfield. His wife, already weakened by **consumption**, stayed with him but died of the disease.

Basic food items were brought to the edge of the village and the villagers left money in a stream or if there was no running water a **plague stone** filled with **vinegar**. The Earl of Devonshire, living a few miles away in Chatsworth House, was a generous benefactor providing food and medical supplies to be delivered to the outskirts of the village. There may have been an ulterior motive in keeping the villagers well fed, but quarantined, a small price to pay for his own good health.

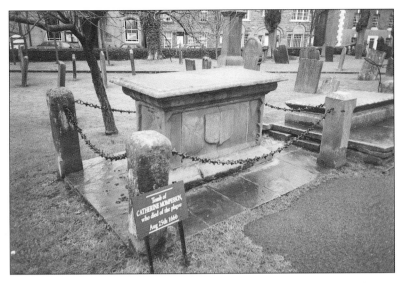

The tomb of Catherine Mompesson in Eyam, Derbyshire. Every year on the last Sunday in August a wreath of flowers is placed on the tomb in memory of her sacrifice in staying to help her husband. William Mompesson wrote of her death, 'My dearest Dear is gone to her eternall rest . . . having made a most happy end: and had she loved herselfe as well as mee, she had fled from the pit of destruction with her sweet infants, and might have p'longed her dayes.'

Mompesson realised the hazard of people congregating in a confined space for worship and preached instead outside in the fresh air standing on a rock. An annual service is held on the last Sunday in August to remember the selflessness and courage of the villagers of Eyam.

EYES. An urban myth persisted until quite recently that having your ears pierced improved your eyesight. Weak eyes or 'dim sight' were cured according to a 1930s home remedy book by bathing the eyes with equal parts of **vinegar**, brandy and cold water.

A cold tea bag on the eye soothed eye strain. See also **ground ivy**.

To heal a 'black eye' a nice juicy raw steak was held on the eye.

In earlier times John Wesley advised in his *Primitive Physic* 2 or 3 drops of rotten **apple** juice to cure 'dull sight' and inflamed eyes. Other problems with the eyes were treated with the astringent

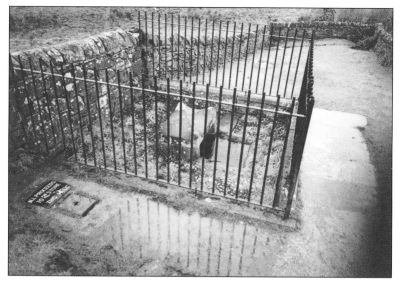

Mompesson's Well on the edge of the village of Eyam in Derbyshire. Basic provisions for the villagers were left at the well as it provided running water to cleanse the money left to pay for them.

plant *Euphrasia* (eyebright) which contains anti-inflammatory properties. Its early use was an example of the **Doctrine of Signatures** as the flower is white, yellow or tinted violet with an orange spot looking like a bleary, bloodshot eye.

There were many industrial processes that caused deteriorating eyesight. In the Black Country chainmakers suffered in later life from heatray cataracts and blindness due to constantly staring into a white hot fire. Other trades like nailmakers, seamstress, miners and those working with lead all suffered eye diseases. In the Black Country rain that fell on Good Friday was collected to treat eye problems.

F

If you wish to be healthy, live on sixpence a day, and earn it.

FAINTING. Tight corsets, hot stuffy rooms, a ladylike sensitivity to horrid sights and shocks, **fever** and **anaemia** were just some of the things to bring on a faint. No Victorian lady was without her smelling salts of **sal volatile** or **hartshorn**, a form of ammonia, and a quick sniff would soon jolt them back into consciousness. Afterwards a glass of port or brandy was a comforting restorative.

FALLING SICKNESS. Another name for **epilepsy**.

FART. As a result of the constant attention to the **bowels** Englishmen were, and some might say still are, particularly affected. A lady belonging to the Women's Institute shared this cheeky little ditty with me after I had given a talk to her members:

> 'A fart is a breeze,
> It gives the belly ease
> It warms up the bedclothes
> And kills off the fleas.'

FASTIN' SPITTLE. Also called 'fasted' and a country expression referring to the first spit of the day. The **saliva** was considered to be stronger on waking up and more effective as a cure when rubbed onto a **stye** or a **wart**. It was also rubbed into the earlobe after ear piercing to speed up the healing.

FATIGUE. An old, surprisingly effective, method of relieving tiredness was to warm the soles of the feet in front of the fire.

FEET. A story from my book *Down the Yorkshire Pan* recounted how Tom 'Tipster', the gentleman who emptied the nightsoil in Nidderdale, North Yorkshire in the 1900s stopped his cart one day and said to a villager, 'My feet are killing me!' He was advised to perhaps try washing them. Next time Tom saw the villager he thanked him and was delighted to be able to say that the advice had worked and his feet were a lot better.

Taking a bath was not always easy when every drop of water had to be heated in the side boiler of the kitchen range and transferred by hand to a tin bath in front of the fire.

An old army trick for overcoming the smell from sweaty feet was to sprinkle **oatmeal** or bran in the socks.

Miners returning home with hot aching feet after a hard day down the pit would 'wee' into a chamber pot and sit soaking their feet in the **urine**.

John Butterworth in his *Practical Medical and Commercial Remedies* of 1897 observed: 'Many people, to the intense annoyance of their neighbours, are much troubled with excessive perspiration of the feet.' To those ever caught downwind of a smelly pair of today's designer footwear – trainers, the problem is still with us. John Butterworth advised washing the feet with a weak solution of permanganate of potash, a powerful and colourful disinfectant. If not dissolved in sufficient water it is likely to leave the feet a lovely pink colour.

FEMALE CONSTITUTION. See also **nervous disorders** and **hysteria**. Women were regarded by male doctors, husbands, fathers and brothers as weak in mind and body as 'Excess sensibility and irritability renders them particularly liable to many distressing affections.'

A Victorian doctor writing in a pamphlet on the 'Physical Effects of Tea' warned: 'The nervous ailments of female constitutions, which are often induced and aggravated by **tea** drinking, in advanced age are apt to terminate in **palsy**. And from a concomitant torpor of the absorbent system of vessels, they also frequently terminate in general **dropsy**.'

Even in the 1930s, by which time they had contributed hugely to the First World War effort, women were still seen as 'the weaker vessel'. A home remedy book listed female complaints as: 'Irregularities, **hysteria**, **headache**, costiveness, loss of appetite, pains and lassitude. The answer according to this book was a dose of **quinine** or **pennyroyal**.

FENNEL. *Foeniculum vulgare*, also known as fenkel. The leaves, roots and seeds have diuretic properties and it was used for centuries in drinks and **infusions** to lose weight. It also relieved spasms and **flatulence**. **Culpepper** recommended it for those who had eaten 'Poisonfull herbs or mushrooms'.

FENNINGS FEVER CURE. Other products were Fennings Little Healers and Fennings Children's Powder, patent remedies used extensively for children cutting their teeth and for all feverish ailments. Made by Alfred Fennings on the Isle of Wight, the medicine was 30% **liquorice** and the rest was potassium chlorate, which had a soothing action on the mucous membranes.

FEVER. A term used in many illnesses when the temperature rises together with shivering, sickness, headaches and extreme tiredness. Not knowing the specific nature of the illness did not stop doctors and family members tackling the fever with gusto.

Eating cooked dove's breast was thought to transfer the coolness of the dove to the patient and overcome the fever.

The fever was treated in many instances with cold bathing, sponging with **vinegar** and in extreme cases a bucket of cold water thrown over the feverish patient. In the 1800s **juniper** berries were chewed to prevent fever and **rosemary** burnt in bedrooms to clear a fever but if a **cobweb** remained in the house the fever would linger on it. When nursing you tried to wash the mouth, nostrils and hands with **vinegar** on leaving the sick room.

See also **beetroot**, **feverfew**, and **tar water**.

FEVERFEW. *Tanacetum parthenium*. A strong smelling, awful tasting herb which grows everywhere in the garden once you make the mistake of accepting the plant as a gift! It is a tonic herb that relieves pain and dilates the blood vessels and was once widely used to reduce **fever**. See also **headache**.

FIGWORT. *Scrophularia nodosa*. Also known as thornwort. A perennial herb found in damp, wet places. **Culpepper** recommended it for the **King's evil** and it was used for centuries to treat skin diseases and inflammation. See also **boils**.

FISH. Children were told to eat their fish as it would give them brains. Recent medical research shows this 'old wives' tale to have some truth in it. Children with dyslexia and attention deficit

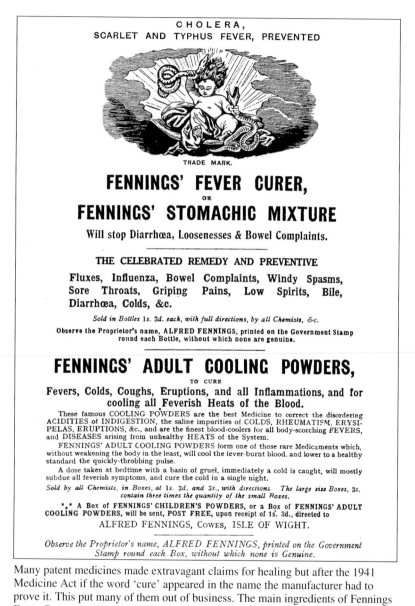

CHOLERA,
SCARLET AND TYPHUS FEVER, PREVENTED

TRADE MARK.

FENNINGS' FEVER CURER,
OR
FENNINGS' STOMACHIC MIXTURE

Will stop Diarrhœa, Loosenesses & Bowel Complaints.

THE CELEBRATED REMEDY AND PREVENTIVE

Fluxes, Influenza, Bowel Complaints, Windy Spasms, Sore Throats, Griping Pains, Low Spirits, Bile, Diarrhœa, Colds, &c.

Sold in Bottles 1s. 3d. *each, with full directions, by all Chemists,* &c.

Observe the Proprietor's name, ALFRED FENNINGS, printed on the Government Stamp round each Bottle, without which none are genuine.

FENNINGS' ADULT COOLING POWDERS,
TO CURE
Fevers, Colds, Coughs, Eruptions, and all Inflammations, and for cooling all Feverish Heats of the Blood.

These famous COOLING POWDERS are the best Medicine to correct the disordering ACIDITIES of INDIGESTION, the saline impurities of COLDS, RHEUMATISM, ERYSIPELAS, ERUPTIONS, &c., and are the finest blood-coolers for all body-scorching FEVERS, and DISEASES arising from unhealthy HEATS of the System.

FENNINGS' ADULT COOLING POWDERS form one of those rare Medicaments which, without weakening the body in the least, will cool the fever-burnt blood, and lower to a healthy standard the quickly-throbbing pulse.

A dose taken at bedtime with a basin of gruel, immediately a cold is caught, will mostly subdue all feverish symptoms, and cure the cold in a single night.

Sold by all Chemists, in Boxes, at 1s. 3d. *and* 3s., *with directions. The large size Boxes,* 3s. *contain three times the quantity of the small Boxes.*

*** A Box of FENNINGS' CHILDREN'S POWDERS, or a Box of FENNINGS' ADULT COOLING POWDERS, will be sent, POST FREE, upon receipt of 1s. 3d., directed to
ALFRED FENNINGS, COWES, ISLE OF WIGHT.

Observe the Proprietor's name, ALFRED FENNINGS, printed on the Government Stamp round each Box, without which none is Genuine.

Many patent medicines made extravagant claims for healing but after the 1941 Medicine Act if the word 'cure' appeared in the name the manufacturer had to prove it. This put many of them out of business. The main ingredients of Fennings Fever Cure were liquorice and potassium chlorate which was also used in fireworks and matches but had disinfectant properties. (By kind permission of the Thackray Museum, Leeds) hyperactive disorder may benefit from taking fish oils and fish has omega-3 series fatty acids which help with a healthy brain function.

Fish is easily digestible and in my childhood if you were ill, whatever the illness, you were given steamed or poached fish – disgusting stuff sitting in a milky liquid, served whether you had a broken ankle or an upset tummy.

Fish was traditionally eaten in Lent but with some suspicion as people thought it gave you **worms**, and large amounts of **tansy** were eaten to get rid of these worms. Even today some people will never touch mackerel for that very reason.

FLANNEL. Old and young were urged to wear flannel next to the skin and ideally it must be coloured red. Given the draughty houses and manual work in all weathers, there was a lot of sense in this. The one drawback was that not everyone washed their piece of flannel regularly. Children could be sewn into undergarments in the autumn and not released from them until the spring.

FLATULENCE. Always seen as a problem. Even in ruder, rougher times a 15th century *Book of Curtesy* warned, 'Beware of thy hinder parts from gun blasting!' Mrs Beeton in her 1861 *Book of Household Management* recommended **olive oil** as a cure. An old almanac published in 1909 believed that 'this complaint is more common in women than men, especially such as are inclined to be hysterical.'

To ease the flatulence either **peppermint** water or a few drops of **ginger** essence could be taken in water or if neither of these were to hand you were advised to drink a glass of hot water. See also **fennel**.

An **infusion** of a small amount of aniseed and cumin in a cup of boiling water was recommended.

Or you could eat charcoal in the form of burnt **toast**.

FLOWERS OF SULPHUR. A fine gritty substance – the deposits of heated crude **sulphur**. See also **sore throat**.

FLUX. From the Latin *fluxus* meaning 'flowing', this refers to an abnormal amount of discharge from any bodily opening. Bloody flux referred to **dysentery**, white flux to the **whites** otherwise known as leucorrhoea.

FOXGLOVE. *Digitalis purpurea*. All parts of the foxglove are highly toxic. William Withering, a physician at the Birmingham General Hospital, discovered in the 1770s that foxglove leaves strengthened and regulated the contractions of the heart. They contain a substance which is the source of digitalis and were used in an **infusion** in the treatment of **dropsy** in folk medicine. As the heart beat stronger the kidneys functioned properly and excreted the excess fluid from the body. By the time William Withering died in 1799, what had long been known by 'the old wives' of Shropshire as foxglove tea, was now recognised as a valuable treatment for failing hearts. A foxglove was carved on his tombstone.

Digitalis poisoning must have been a frequent occurrence. Even as recently as the 1930s home remedy books recommended its use as a home medicine. 'Foxglove is such an active medicine that it will cure when all other remedies fail, and will completely restore beyond expectations . . . in the most hopeless case it will prolong life, and when death takes place whilst under its influence it is often without pain or struggle. Not more than half a teaspoonful of the dried leaf rubbed to powder to be used in one day to half a pint of boiling water.'

FRACTIOUS BABIES. See **bicarbonate of soda**.

FRECKLES. Hardly an illness but some in pursuit of a flawless white face got in quite a tizz about them. In Elizabethan times you were advised to smear the face with the sap of a birch tree. However, the advice by the late 1800s from *The Lady's World* was far more dangerous. 'In the Eastern countries the ladies of the seraglio are said to value highly a wash known as Oriental Cosmetic for the purpose of removing freckles. The basis of this wash has been found to be perchloride of mercury.'

FRIARS' BALSAM. A compound tincture of benzoin or **benjamin**, a gum resin from a species of laurel. The mixture was known by

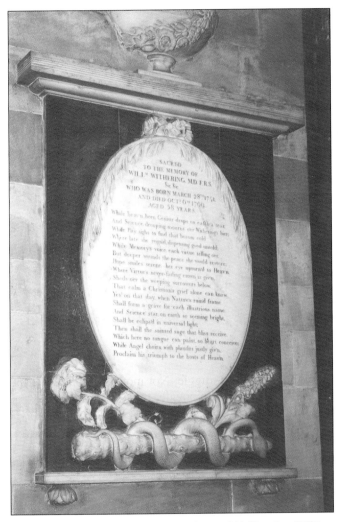

The magnificent memorial stone in Edgbaston Old Church to William Withering (1741–1799) who discovered the medical value of the foxglove. Anyone who has ever benefited from his discovery might well echo the full blown language of the day, 'While heav'n born Genius drops on earth a tear, And Science drooping mourns o'er Withering's bier.' Interesting imagery with the foxglove carving and the staff of Asclepius, the Greek god of medicine, with the serpent coiled around it, known world wide as the symbol of medicine. (Photograph Linda Ibbetson-Price by kind permission of the Vicar of Edgbaston The Reverend Edward D. Coombes)

several names; Jesuits' Drops, Commander's Balsam and Traumatic Balsam. No one is sure how it came by the name Friars' but anything with the name Jesuit attached to it was highly unpopular in the late 1600s. By the early 1700s it was known as Friars' Balsam.

Inhaling Friars' Balsam in a pint of boiling water with a towel over the head was a stock cure for a **cold**; others took 2 drops on a lump of sugar. It could also be used on abrasions.

FROG SPAWN. An 18th century North Country remedy recommended washing in water containing frog spawn to reduce redness and for a clear, healthy skin.

FRUITS THAT CURE DISEASES. An interesting list from a 1930s home remedy book and one with which we cannot argue, even if disputing quite such generous claims for the fruit listed.

'Of all forms of diet none are so curative as fruits and of these probably the **apple** is king. A French physician has lately discovered that the bacillus of **typhoid** lives but a short time in apple juice. Of fruit generally, as remedial agents, it may be said that sloes contain phosphates which are of benefit for bloodlessness and brain fag; mulberries, cherries and strawberries relieve **gout** and **rheumatism**; gooseberries correct the ill-effects of too rich foods and red and white currants purify the blood. Baked bananas are among the most easily digested foods.'

FULLER'S EARTH. *Aluminium silicate.* The smooth grey powder was thought to be helpful for chafings and sores and as a **poultice** for inflamed eyes. More recently in the early 1960s it was used by some of us as a cheap face pack for a spotty teenage skin.

FUNDAMENT. An old name for the anus. Young children can sometimes suffer a prolapse or protrusion of the rectum. John Wesley in his *Primitive Physic* advised pushing it back either with a cloth 'covered thick with Brick Dust,' or 'Boil a handful of Red Rose Leaves in a quart (*sic*) of a pint of red wine; Dip a cloth in it, and apply it as hot as can be borne.'

He also thought this would work on 'A Falling down of the **womb**'.

G

When out of sorts, give nature a chance.

GANGLION. A harmless swelling, usually found on the back of the wrist. Traditionally dealt with by hitting it with the heavy old family Bible.

GARLIC. *Allium sativum*. The many health-giving properties of garlic are now well known and there is no shortage of products in health food shops. It has important antiseptic properties, reduces **fever** and aids digestion.

It was introduced to Britain by the Romans but with our usual distrust of anything 'foreign', we failed to latch on to its culinary and medical uses. Instead we hung it on our front doors to guard against witches.

John Wesley in *Primitive Physic* recommended for **rheumatism,** 'Soaking 7 cloves of garlic in half a pint of white wine and drink it lying down'.

See also **corns**.

GATHERING. Another name for an **abscess** or **whitlow** at the base of a fingernail. Dipping the finger in scalding water in the early stages of the gathering was one, painful, way of dealing with it.

GENTIAN VIOLET. A dye derived from methane and painted onto a shaved head for the highly infectious impetigo. It is a good antiseptic and was also used on **burns**.

GERARD. John Gerard (1545–1612) born in Nantwich, Cheshire. He served a 7 years apprenticeship in London as a **barber-surgeon** but became increasingly interested in his garden near Holborn and studying the medicinal properties of the plants he was growing there. His *Herball*, published in 1597, listed over 1,000 species and became hugely popular and influential in the medicine of the day.

GIN. At one time known as 'Mother's Ruin' or 'Dutch Courage'. Gin was first invented by a Dutch Professor of Medicine who distilled maize, malt and rye with **juniper** berries. In Holland it was called Geneva Gin, a corruption from the French word for juniper 'genièvre'. At first it was considered a medicine and Victorian mothers used a drop in the bottle, to get the baby to nod off. Unscrupulous childminders drugged whole nurseries of babies in order to get some peace and the babies passed their days in an alcohol induced sleep.

Gin was cheap, easily available and often led to squalid addiction. The effects on the poor alarmed social reformers. George Cruikshank (1792–1878) the painter and illustrator became an ardent teetotaller in 1847, the same year he published *The Bottle*. His series of drawings showed a happy, prosperous family enjoying a first 'nip', followed then by a dark descent into penury, murder and madness. 'From the bar of the Gin Shop to the Bar of the Old Bailey It Is But One Step!' The final picture in the sequence shows the daughter, 'Homeless, Deserted, Destitute and Gin Mad', throwing herself off a bridge. These powerful images helped fuel the growing popularity of the Temperence movement.

However, some still saw gin as a medicine. Gin and hot water sweetened with a little sugar was a favourite remedy for 'period pains'. Others went a little further and drank neat gin while taking a hot bath as an **abortificant**.

In the 1930s and 40s washing a child's hair in gin was said to kill head lice but it had to be Geneva gin for some reason.

Even today there is a popular home remedy using gin for **arthritis** and some find it helpful for the skin complaint psoriasis. Empty a small box of sultanas into a container and pour over enough neat gin to cover. Let it stand until the sultanas have absorbed the gin and eat 9 sultanas a day.

A teacher giving a lesson to a class of 9 and 10 year olds on the dangers of alcohol put before the class an empty glass beaker. Into this he poured some neat gin followed by a live worm. Not unexpectedly the worm died and the teacher turned to the children and said 'Now what does this teach us about alcohol?' And a bright lad from the back put his hand up and said, 'Please sir, if you've got worms – drink gin.'

GINGER. The root of the *Zingiber officinale*. It is a warming **carminative** herb that increases perspiration, stimulates the circulation and helps with digestion.

We now know that the volatile oils in ginger help reduce motion sickness but in the past all we knew was that for sea or travel sickness of any sort, you ate a couple of ginger biscuits.

Ginger increases the production of saliva and will help with a **sore throat** or dry **cough**.

Chewing a piece of ginger when visiting a sickroom was believed to keep you clear of contagion.

A teaspoonful of ginger tincture would help in cases of **flatulence** and was added to many homemade **aperients, purgatives** and patent medicines.

GLAUBER'S SALTS. Sulphate of soda, a strong **purgative** originally named after J. R. Glauber, a German chemist.

GOITRE. Iodine helps form the thyroid hormone which controls the metabolism. Too little thyroid hormone leads to hypothyroidism, signified by an unsightly swelling on the front of the neck. It was caused by a lack of iodine in drinking water and deep valleys in mountainous areas were particularly affected. Once known as Derbyshire Neck as it was common in the Peak District.

The illness was known for centuries but not understood and it was treated in the same way as the **King's evil**. Eating seaweed, which is high in **iodine**, was known to have some effect but if you lived in a remote hill area you were very far from the sea and any source of seaweed.

It was an illness affecting mostly women and a retired doctor remembered as a young man it was a common sight to see women hugely disfigured by these swellings.

GOLDEN ROD. *Solidago virgaurea*. This plant has many medicinal properties including diuretic, expectorant and anti-inflammatory and can help in relaxing spasms. See also **morning sickness**.

It was used extensively in the Middle Ages for **wounds**. A home remedy was to bind a deep wound with strips of cotton soaked in a solution of golden rod.

GOOSE GREASE. The huge amount of goose fat coming out of the bird while cooking was lovingly collected and hoarded in earthenware pots. Sometimes it was mixed with **camphor**. Goose grease was rubbed onto the chest and back for **coughs, colds** and **bronchitis**. It was a powerful insulator of heat and for good measure a layer of **brown paper** or red **flannel** was added underneath a vest or liberty bodice.

Goose fat was mixed with gorse flowers to make an ointment, known as Yorkshire Goose Salve, for healing the sore hands of Whitby fishermen.

GOUT. An illness occurring mostly in men, it once was seen as the result of too much port and fine living. An excess of uric-acid salts collects in the joints leading to painful swelling and redness. The caricature figure associated with gout is the old aristocrat, with his foot swathed in bandages resting on a footstool, being served another glass of port by his butler. Gout was not seen as all bad as Dr Samuel Johnson (1709–84), the great lexicographer, was not alone in believing that having gout prevented you from catching anything worse.

John Wesley in his *Primitive Physic* knew the belief of gout as a prophylactic but warned against it, 'Regard not them who say, The Gout ought not to be cured.' He advised rubbing the affected part in warm treacle and then binding on some **flannel**.

The Family Physician of 1794 recommended the highly unlikely cure of: 'Take frequently a cup of strong **negus** or a glass of generous wine.'

An old Northamptonshire cure recommended eating a dozen walnuts a day.

Strawberries were thought helpful in treating gout as was the external application of dried **sage** leaves or **ground elder** in a **poultice**.

See also **Bath**.

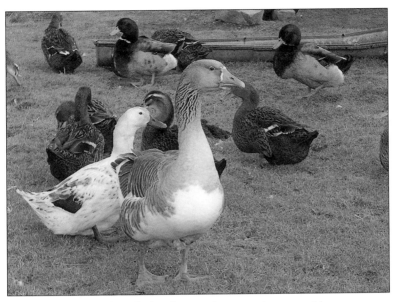

What a useful bird! After enjoying the meat from a roast goose nothing was wasted. Goose grease was kept in stone jars for rubbing on and homemade ointments, a wing made a good chimney brush and the feathers stuffed eiderdowns and pillows. They even make good 'guard dogs' and can be very protective of their property. (Photograph Sylvia Turner)

GRAVEL. The small, rough calculi or sediment in the kidney or bladder. Like **bladder stones** it was a common problem in the past.

John Wesley advised, 'Eat largely of Spinach.'

In 1848 *The New London Cookery and Complete Domestic Guide* by 'A Lady' advised, 'Pour a quart of boiling water onto a spoonful each of **honey** and **oatmeal**, stir well, allow to cool and drink half on going to bed and the other half in the morning.'

This splendid book contained 'The Complete Guide on the Principles of Frugality, Comfort and Elegance, including the Art of Carving and the most approved method of setting out a table', together with 'The Instructions for Preserving Health and Attaining Old Age'. Could today's glamorous or laddish TV cooks produce such a book?

It was still a problem in the 1930s when drinking a tea made from **agrimony** sweetened with sugar together with abstaining from 'high living' was seen as the answer.

GREGORY POWDER. A family favourite bought from the chemist and used as a **purgative**. Pale yellow in colour it contained **rhubarb**, magnesia and **ginger**.

GRIPPE. An old name for **influenza**.

GROCERS' ITCH. The once familiar blue bags of sugar in the grocer's shop presented a problem for the person 'bagging' it up. Raw sugar, more often than not, contained colonies of the sugar mite *Acarus sacchari*. The mite burrowed under the fingernails, producing an irritating pustular disease called 'Grocer's itch'. According to *The Practical Grocer* of 1905 it was estimated that there were as many as 100,000 acari present in each pound of sugar.

The itch was cured by using **sulphur**.

GROUND ELDER. *Aegopodium podagraria*. Also known as goutweed. A keen gardener will view ground elder with loathing. It advances at a tremendous rate, smothering everything before it and if when you pull it up you leave just a tiny bit of root, it continues with renewed vigour.

The Romans introduced the plant to this country as they ate the leaves as a vegetable. In the Middle Ages the monks used it for its diuretic and anti-inflammatory medicinal properties. The leaves were used in a **poultice** for **gout** and **stings**.

GROUND IVY. *Glechoma hederacea*. Known in country areas as Robin-run-in-hedge and by the older name of alehoof as before hops were introduced here in the 16th century it was used in brewing.

An **infusion** of the leaves was made into a tea called 'gill tea' from the French 'guiller', to ferment ale and was given in the treatment of **coughs** and **consumption**. The plant has expectorant and diuretic properties and acts as a tonic and for this reason was once used in the treatment of **tuberculosis** and **typhus**.

According to the 1895 **commonplace book** belonging to the Wensleydale farmer Edward Brown it was good for 'Anyone troubled with their water'.

The juice of the leaves, which are rich in vitamin C, was thought to cure **jaundice** and **eczema** and the leaves were sold on the streets of London for people to make a lotion for sore and inflamed **eyes**. The dried leaves were also crushed and used as a snuff to cure a **headache**.

This little plant regarded as a weed and found at the bottom of most hedgerows, is now overlooked but at one time it was used to treat practically anything. See also **wounds**.

GROUNDSEL. *Senecio vulgaris*. A bitter and astringent diuretic herb once used for any **menstrual** problems and the **menopause** but now considered unsafe.

John Wesley in his *Primitive Physic* recommended it as a cure for **ague**: 'Take a handful of groundsel, shred it small, put it into a paper bag 4 inches square, pricking that side which is next to the skin full of holes. Cover this with a thin linen, and wear it on the pit of the stomach.'

In Somerset they used groundsel in a **poultice** to clear an **abscess**.

GUINNESS. For many years this popular drink had an almost mythical status as in people's minds it was a readily accessible remedy for most illnesses. The brewery, founded in 1759, did nothing to promote this idea, indeed the first Lord Iveagh, Edward Cecil Guinness, who governed the brewery from 1876 to 1927, was positively opposed to any form of advertising. He firmly believed that Guinness must sell on the purity of its ingedients; malt, roasted barley, hops, yeast and water.

Beer was considered a good clean drink, unlike the wicked **gin** and the 'word on the street' was that Guinness was good for you. Many looked on a small glass a day, especially when taken after dinner, as a general tonic with some strong recuperative properties.

Advertising Guinness started in 1927 and by 1929 the company was receiving countless testimonials:

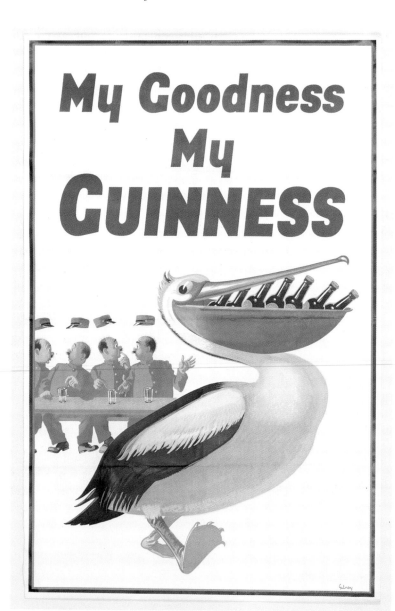

A 1939 poster for Guinness by the artist J. Gilroy. (By kind permission of the Guinness Archives)

From Great Yarmouth – 'It has been meat and drink to me for many years and as a hypnotic and balm for my tired and worn out nerves.'

From Harrow – 'I have noticed that women who take stout never seem to have trouble with their milk – I insist on my wife taking a small glass daily.'

From St Helens – 'I was considerably run down after my war service and the results of wounds and suffered from wasting and insomnia. A bottle of Guinness each night was taken until I made steady progress and now I am in full mental and physical vigour.'

A doctor writing from Eastbourne, unwittingly painted a picture of life in that town between the two World Wars. ' My practice consists largely of neurotic and neurasthenic patients, eg. overworked and underfed clergy, missionaries, shop assistants and independent spinsters approaching or enduring the climateric. Now these patients, I find, respond very readily to the treatment of fresh air, rest, copious good food and a sedative, and for the latter my practice is as a rule to prescribe Guinness.'

Other conditions for which people believed a drop of Guinness would do you good were **boils**, **consumption**, **constipation**, **sea sickness** . . . and even golf! '. . . After a light luncheon and a bottle of Guinness . . . my game is much improved!'

GYPSIES. Some travelling gypsies in the 17th and 18th centuries performed the same services as the **barber-surgeons**. Using their caravans, like a mobile operating theatre, they were quite skilled at performing minor procedures; cutting out a cyst, pulling a tooth or bone setting. They were believed to be especially gifted at **wart** charming. See also **eczema**.

H

The window opened more would keep doctor's wealth from the door.

HARROGATE. Once regarded as the 'Queen of Inland Watering Places'. A chalybeate or iron spring was first dicovered in 1571 by William Slingsby of Bilton Park. The Tewitt Well was promoted as having medicinal properties and the discovery of further wells put Harrogate on the map. Michael Stanhope, writing in 1632, was not happy with the class of visitor, describing the springs as, 'Being used by the vulgar sort [where] they wash their soares and cleanse their besmeared clouths, where diverse after dippe their cups to drinke.'

With the discovery in 1695 of the strong saline **sulphur** well, aptly called The Stinking Spaw, health tourism flourished with

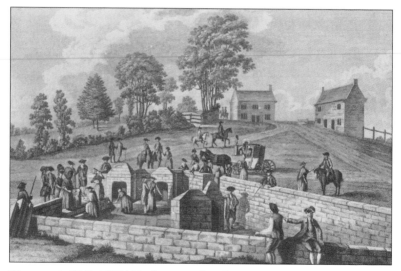

'Harrowgate Wells 1772.' The horses preferred to stay at a distance from the well heads because of the strong sulphur smell. A Dr. Deane in 1626 claimed that the Harrogate waters 'Cheereth and reviveth the spirits, strengtheneth the stomach, causeth good and quick appetite and furthereth digestion.'(By kind permission of Harrogate Museums and Art Gallery Service)

hotels, lodging houses and shops all there to provide a comfortable stay and take your money.

In the late 17th and 18th centuries drinking 2 pints a day of the foul smelling water was considered good for you. The smell was such that horses refused to go near the well.

A recommendation written in 1875 advised that drinking the water would 'Prove highly beneficial in most forms of **indigestion** with its usual accompaniments: **constipation**, **flatulence** and acidity; all cases of functional disorders of the **liver**, even when that organ has undergone material organic changes especially those resulting from free living and inactive habits, combined with excess of alcohol.'

Besides drinking the waters you also bathed in them for the relief of **rheumatism**, **gout**, skin diseases and general well being. Luxurious bathing establishments were built to cater for royalty, politicians, celebrities and the great and the good. The Royal Baths, which opened in 1897, offered the most advanced hydrotherapy to match any European **spa** town. There were 77 treatments on offer including the oddly named Carbonic Acid Bath, Vichy douches, the Sitz Bath and a sumptuous Turkish Bath.

At the end of your stay you took home a small tin of Harrogate Health Salts. The locals spent many hours boiling sulphur water to extract the salts. A half teaspoon in cold water was recommended for all forms of **indigestion**, **rheumatism** and the usual old favourites, **constipation** and **flatulence**.

HARTSHORN. An old name for **sal volatile** used for sniffing by Victorian ladies when about to suffer a **fainting** attack. The horn from a hart, a male deer aged over 5 years, was once used as the main source of ammonia.

HAWKWEED. *Hieracium pilosella*. Also known as mouse ear grass. This plant was known to **Culpepper** and was recognised even then as having expectorant properties. In parts of North Kent, especially the more industrial, the water in which hawkweed had been boiled was drunk as a cure for **whooping cough**.

HAWTHORN. *Crataegus laevigata*. Also known as may, when it flowers. The leaves were once eaten by country people between 2 slices of bread giving rise to the other name of 'bread and cheese'. The berries have been used since the Middle Ages as a tonic for an ageing and strained heart.

Quite recently I was told of someone, living on a farm on the outskirts of Bradford, who had lived to be over 100. Her grand-daughter explained grandma's longevity as due to a daily medicinal drop of hawthorn berry juice. Her method was to pick ripe red hawthorn berries, put them in a bottle and cover with brandy. The liquid was left until it became red when she took 2 or 3 drops on a sugar cube every day. Modern day medicine acknowledges what grandma already knew, that the berries enlarge the coronary vessels, strengthen the heart and can control hypertension.

The hawthorn also has its grim side for there are many legends and most of them negative. Never bring hawthorn blossom indoors or someone you love will die that year, never sit under a hawthorn hedge as the fairies will claim you, and never destroy or cut a hawthorn hedge or something awful will occur.

This reputation for dark happenings is linked with the **Black Death**. After the disease wiped out many villages in the 14th century, hawthorn bushes sprang up in the depopulated and increasingly desolate countryside. The blossom contains a chemical which is very like the smell of putrefaction and it was said resembled the odour of London during the **bubonic plague** of 1665.

HAZLENUT. An old country superstition believed that carrying a double hazelnut in your pocket meant you would never suffer from **toothache**. The double hazelnut was also a good luck symbol for a happy marriage.

HEADACHE. See also **migraine**. Edwardian doctors believed that the root cause of a headache was to be found in '**constipation** together with close and prolonged confinement in overheated and badly ventilated rooms', and also sitting with your legs crossed.

In the 1930s a cure for a headache was a little **nutmeg** taken in water. 'Why suffer?' said the home remedy book and if this failed there was always the whisky remedy: One thimbleful of whisky rubbed onto the hands and then held to the nose – breathe deeply.

The sniffing of a substance with a powerful smell was a well known cure and included brandy, **camphorated oil**, **horseradish**, **lavender**, lemon zest, smelling salts, snuff and **vinegar**.

If none of these were to hand you made a pot of tea, lifted the lid and held your forehead over the steam. See also **ground ivy**.

You were recommended to eat the boiled leaves of **feverfew** as a vegetable or raw in a sandwich. See also **Beecham's pills**.

The common sense option of keeping the head cool was achieved by placing either a **cabbage** or lettuce leaf in your hat. But John Wesley's idea in *Primitive Physic* might not be to everyone's liking: 'Order a tea-kettle of cold water to be poured on your head every morning in a slender stream.'

On the other hand sitting with your feet in warm water was a cheap cure, ideally for 15 minutes before going to bed.

All the above were preferable to the advice on how to cure a headache given by Maximilian Hazlemore in 1794, very much a man of his time: 'The patient may be bled in the jugular vein. **Cupping** also or the application of **leeches** to the temples and behind the ears. Afterwards a blistering **plaster** may be applied to the neck, behind the ears or to any part of the head that is most affected – for some cases it will be proper to **blister** the whole head.' The words that come to mind are 'sledgehammer' and 'nut'.

HEAD LICE. See **nits**.

HEARTBURN. A simple, cheap remedy from the Black Country was to take a well washed lump of coal and suck it.

A pleasant soothing cure from Northumberland mixed the juice of a **lemon** with a little water, and half a teaspoon of **bicarbonate of soda**.

John Wesley in his *Primitive Physic* had a more complicated, if unlikely, remedy: 'Take 6 Almonds add 12 raw Peas, and eat them together.'

See also **chamomile**.

HEART DISEASE. Little could be done but a 1930s home remedy book advised a tablespoon of whisky in a little milk. See also **dropsy**, **foxglove** and **hawthorn**.

HEDGE GARLIC. *Alliaria petiolata*. Also known as garlic mustard or Jack-by-the-hedge. Its pungent flavour meant it was used in sauces for fish or boiled mutton and gave rise to its other name – sauce alone. It has medicinal healing and antiseptic properties and the dried leaves taken like snuff were said to 'clear the head' and calm those suffering from **hysteria** thereby preventing, it was thought, their further descent into mental illness.

HENBANE. *Hyoscyamus niger.* A highly poisonous plant, known since ancient times and always a favourite with poisoners. In Shakespeare's *Hamlet* his father was killed by henbane poured into his ear. The plant has narcotic, sedative and pain killing properties and it was used in Victorian times in the treatment of **migraine**.

HERB ROBERT. *Geranium robertianum*. Also known as stinking Bob. Geraniums are high in tannins with astringent and healing properties. It was used in a **poultice** on painful **joints**.

Like the **hawthorn** it was surrounded by myth and shares with that plant a rather nasty fetid smell, hence the alternative name. Used since the Middle Ages for staunching bleeding and healing **wounds**, it is associated in folklore with magic.

HEROIC. A word referring to the large doses (heroic doses) of often dangerous drugs together with the savage **blood-letting** and **purging** that were the standard medical procedures (heroic medicine) right up to the middle of the 19th century. Home remedies were a very attractive alternative.

HERNIA. See **rupture**.

HICCUP. Alternative spelling Hiccough. Everyone can offer a favourite cure for a bout of hiccups.

Breathe into a brown paper bag 20 times.

Hold your breath and count mentally to 20.

Drink lemon juice or vinegar.

Drink a glass of water from the opposite side of the glass.

Swallow a mouthful of water whilst holding the mouth tightly shut and holding your ears.

Make yourself sneeze with a little pepper.

Eat some **ginger**.

Stand on your head (this cure is only available to the fit and agile).

From the Black Country a simple idea for a cure: hold one arm outstretched level with the shoulder until the hiccups subside, using the left arm if you are right handed and vice versa.

And finally . . ask someone to give you a fright!

HOARSENESS. A pleasant remedy from an old Yorkshire railwayman. Bake a **lemon** as you would an apple and squeeze a little of the thickened and hot juice onto a lump of sugar and take frequently.

A revolting remedy from a 1920s home remedy book advised you to sip hot milk boiled with a little suet.

John Wesley in his *Primitive Physic* offered the unlikely suggestion of: 'Rubbing the soles of the feet before the fire with **garlic** and lard well beaten together. The hoarseness will be gone next day.'

HONEY. Made by bees from nectar and stored in their hives or nests, honey has always been valued and especially today by those interested in alternative medicine. Many swear that a spoonful a day will lead to a long and healthy life. With a high concentration of natural sugars it has been used as a sweetener since ancient times. Honey was recognised for its healing, soothing and anti-inflammatory properties and used to heal **burns**, **chapped hands** and lips, **cuts**, leg **ulcers** and in a **poultice** to heal **boils**.

A further remedy from the Midlands, in particular the Black Country, showed that honey rubbed gently onto a splinter would draw it out or 'fetch' it.

Honey was added to homemade **cough medicines** where its soothing sweetness would have been a great comfort.

HOPS. Grown in the Kent hopfields and used in making beer. Hops and carraway seeds made into a tea were said to restore the appetite and to promote a cheerful mind.

A 1930s home remedy book thought they were invaluable for good health. Not as beer but a quarter of an ounce of hops, a teaspoonful of **Epsom salts** and a pint of boiling water and a wineglassful taken in the morning 'will not only restore, but will keep anyone in the best of health at little expense'. In other words – a **purgative**.

Country people have long believed that a pillow filled with hops would soothe a troubled mind and promote sleep. For a really 'knockout' mixture fill a pillow with 75 hops, some **lavender, rosemary, southernwood** and **tansy**.

HOREHOUND. *Marrubium vulgare*. Also known as white horehound. A bitter aromatic herb first used as a cough medicine by the Egyptians. It has sedative properties which may explain why it was once used in the treatment of **epilepsy**.

HORSERADISH. *Armoracia rusticana*. The name horse attached to a name meant large, strong or coarse. For those who like a hot horseradish as an accompaniment to their roast beef the stronger the better as it is a digestive stimulant. See also **alcoholism, headache** and **lethargy**.

A horseradish **poultice** was thought to relieve **rheumatism**.

HOT FOMENTATION. A home medical procedure once used extensively to draw the pus out of a **boil**. Drop 2-inch squares of lint in a pan of boiling water. Lift out on the end of a wooden spoon, and using a towel for protection, wring out until almost dry. Place lint onto the boil and hold with a pad of cotton wool to keep the heat in. Do this about 10 times every morning and evening.

HOUSELEEK. *Sempervivum tectorum*. The plant contains tannins and was known for its healing properties. John Wesley in *Primitive Physic* recommended a houseleek rubbed onto a **cut** and to this day some people declare there is nothing finer.

The houseleek cut in two and rubbed on the affected skin was a well known cure for **ringworm** and **warts**.

The Romans used the houseleek as a magic charm, planting one on the roof, in the belief that the house would never be struck by lightning.

HOUSEMAID'S KNEE. Another name for bursitis. A chronic inflammation of the bursa in front of the kneecap as a result of too much kneeling. This very painful complaint could be put right by rest; not an option for a poor Victorian housemaid. Miners also suffered similarly from 'miner's knee'. An old remedy from Northumberland used bundles of **marshmallow** leaves and stalks, boiled to a pulp and when slightly cooled strapped to the knee as a **poultice** overnight.

HUMOURS. For good health the Greeks thought the body needed to be 'balanced' and this theory lived on for centuries. It partly explains all the purging and bleeding that went on in medicine. According to the Greek physician Hippocrates (c460–c357 BC), known as the Father of Medicine, the four vital life forces were blood, phlegm, black bile and yellow bile. If one of them became 'unbalanced' you needed to have some bodily fluid drawn off.

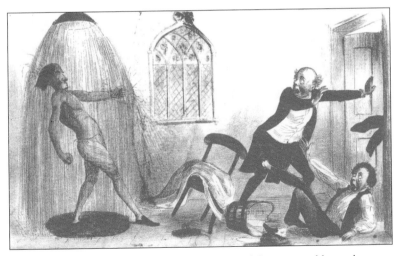

'The Hydropathist' or just one of the many strange sights you would see when taking a water cure. From a humorous Victorian booklet *The Sure Water Cure* price 5/- by Messrs Fores of Picadilly. (By kind permission of Harrogate Museums and Art Gallery Service)

HYSSOP. *Hyssopus officinalis*. The Greeks and Romans knew of the powerful properties of hyssop and it was used extensively in an **infusion** for stomach and chest complaints and as a cleansing herb. Oil of hyssop is particularly powerful and can bring on muscular spasms. John Wesley in *Primitve Physic* recommended it placed in the ear for **earache**.

HYSTERIA. Seen as part of the **female constitution** and as an old Northampton doctor once put it, 'Slam the door loudly when making your exit.' *Family Medical Adviser* written in 1866 had a different approach. 'Hysteria is a disease to which females are often subject. In cases of sudden attack put the feet at once into warm water.' If this did not work the male writer went on to advise loosening the stays and giving an **enema**.

A way of dealing with someone having an attack was to startle or frighten them out of the hysterics. This could be done, somewhat unsympathetically, by slapping the face, throwing cold water at them or putting pepper under the nose to make them sneeze. See also **lady's slipper**.

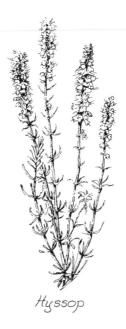

Hyssop

I

More people are slain by late suppers than by the sword.

ILKLEY. This prosperous small town in North Yorkshire became the haunt of the rich and famous when, in the 1849s, its spring waters were found to have medicinal properties. It never rivalled **Harrogate** but it was a popular inland holiday resort with fresh air straight off Ilkley Moor guaranteed to put colour into a city dweller's cheeks.

Its heyday as a centre for hydrotherapy lasted to 1870 but sadly the town's reputation for restoring health suffered a setback when one of its most prominent doctors was discovered to have been the lover of a lady who had scandalised Victorian society by poisoning her husband.

The rousing Yorkshire anthem 'On Ilkla Mooar baht 'at', still sung with gusto by proud Yorkshire people everywhere, is in fact a health warning! Those who go onto the moor without a hat, to do some courting, will undoubtedly catch 'thee deeath of cold'.

INDIAN BRANDEE. A popular tonic patent medicine from the late 1800s through to the early 1900s which had nothing to do with brandy – hence the spelling. An American product with the name Indian referring to the Native Americans, who probably had nothing to do with the recipe. The name was a marketing idea to make customers think it was an age old medicine used by a people in touch with nature. It was a tonic used for digestive problems and contained spirit of **nitre**, **rhubarb** and maple syrup.

INDIGESTION. Many old remedies contained bismuth which was readily obtained and has a sedative action on painful conditions of the **bowels** and stomach. A typical homemade remedy contained ingredients that soothed the **heartburn** and indigestion brought on by fatty, rich foods.

Mix 1 dram of bismuth, 2 teaspoons of **bicarbonate of soda**, 20 drops of **peppermint** esssence. Put in a medicine bottle and fill up with water.

After a heavy meal drink an **infusion** of **sage**.

Victorians knew the value of regular meals and chewing their food slowly. For those able to spare the time a regular nap after lunch was regarded as an essential aid to digestion. The unctuous rogue Mr Pecksniff in Charles Dickens' *Martin Chuzzlewit* summed up the Victorian view of a good digestive action: 'The process of digestion, as I have been informed by anatomical friends, is one of the most wonderful works of nature. I do not know how it may be with others, but it is a great satisfaction to me to know, when regaling on my humble fare, that I am putting in motion the most beautiful machinery with which we have any acquaintance. I really feel at such times as if I was doing a public service.'

See also **Beecham's pills**, **olive oil** and **water**.

INFECTION. To avoid infection while visiting or nursing the sick it was recommended that you smoke a cigarette while near the patient. Other tips from a 1930s home remedy book advised you not to swallow your spittle, always wash with **vinegar**, and use ground **coffee** as snuff.

INFLAMMATION. The painful swelling of body tissues characterised by heat and redness as a result of an infection or injury. The blood supply is increased to the area and the white blood corpuscles attack the bacteria causing the infection. **Turpentine** was used to reduce the redness but probably had an effect in cleansing the skin.

A **tincture** made from the flowers of the **marigold** was an ancient remedy to reduce inflammation and aid the healing process.

INFLUENZA. Once known as Grippe, the English Sweat or Sweating Sickness. The term influenza was first used in this country in 1743 but the illness is thought to have been around since 400 BC. Epidemics swept through the British Isles during the 19th century but the greatest pandemic from February 1918 to January 1919 killed over 25 million worldwide.

Families were orphaned, parents watched helplessly while children, already weakened through poverty, died quickly, quite well one day – dead the next. Communities ground to a halt; there were shortages of coal and gas, schools shut down, hospitals could not cope, trains did not run and sanitary services, such as the emptying of earth closets in towns, ceased.

War censorship meant that the full effects of the pandemic was not reported. However Spain was neutral and reports in the newspapers there gave rise to the name 'Spanish 'Flu' or 'The Spanish Lady'.

Influenza is caused by a virus and death came from broncho-pneumonia for which there was no effective cure. In vain people applied a **bread poultice** to the chest and back to relieve the pain felt on breathing and filled the kitchen with steam from boiling water in saucepans and kettles. **Dover Powder** was given as a sedative and for pain relief. More people died in those few months in this country of influenza than in the whole of the First World War.

INFUSION. A method of soaking in order to extract flavour or other properties: we do this every time we make a cup of tea. For herbal remedies pour 1 pint (600ml) of boiling water onto 1 ounce (25g) of dried herbs or 2 ounces (50g) if using fresh. Cover and leave for 5 to 10 minutes, then strain and drink in the manner of tea.

INSOMNIA. See **sleeplessness** and **bread**.

INVALID. For many being an invalid was a way of life; they could be in a chronic state of ill health from cradle to grave. Death was very real to everyone, spoken of openly, acknowledged, in some cases even welcomed. Infant mortality touched every family, rich or poor – money could not buy good health. Women suffered ill health brought on by too many pregnancies. Men were disabled through industrial accidents and diseases leaving them sick and unable to work.

Yet there was still a feeling that keeping cheerful and busy was a great healer. 'Hints for the Sick Room' written in 1915 offered bracing words, 'Advice to an Invalid – Always set your face firmly towards health. Say that you are better when people enquire; the very declaration will assist in making you feel so. Persistent good cheer and hopefulness are remedial agents very hard to defeat in the conflict between illness and health. . . Work is the best of safeguards, and the surest escape-valve for bodily distress.'

A **low diet** was an essential part of recovery; **calf's foot jelly** was never far away. Home remedy books always had a recipe to tempt the invalid.

Egg Snow for Invalids

Beat together 1 tablespoon of milk, sugar, orange or **lemon** juice. Beat the white of an egg and stir into the mixture.

Calf's foot jelly or egg snow – I know which I would have preferred.

IODINE. A non-metallic element found in seaweed. Painted on the skin, as for swollen glands, it coloured the skin dark brown. See also **toothache**.

Tincture of iodine, once widely used, is no longer available as taken in large doses it is a violent poison. Externally it was used as an antiseptic and dabbed onto a graze; the intense pain it caused brought tears to the eyes.

Iodine lockets were sewn into the clothes right up to the Second World War to prevent **scarlet fever**. See also **goitre**.

IPECACUANHA. Shortened to ipecac and a popular ingredient in home treatments of a **cough** or **cold**. It is the root of the Brazilian shrub *Cephaelis ipecacuanha*. In large doses it causes vomiting but in smaller doses is a gentle stimulant to the respiratory passages and liquifies the thick mucous in chest infections. It was an ingredient in the popular **Dover Powder**.

ITCH. John Wesley in his *Primitive Physic* was unspecific as to the kind of itch and on what part of the body but he may have meant **scabies**. He advised washing the parts affected in strong rum and 'steep a shirt for half an hour in a quart of water mixt with half an ounce of powdered **brimstone**. Dry it slowly and wear it 5 or 6 days.'

IVY. *Hedera helix*. All parts of the ivy are poisonous but that did not stop our ancestors. It was believed the top side of the leaf had healing properties and the underside would draw out infection.

Ivy berry vinegar was a popular remedy for the **bubonic plague** and was used in the Great Plague of London 1665.

A **decoction** from the berries was said to cure **rheumatism**; however, too many berries and you were in serious trouble.

Within living memory a Yorkshire cure for 'gowly' (sticky) eyes was boiling young ivy leaves in water and the eyes bathed in the weak, warm solution. This was seen to be very soothing in cases of **measles**.

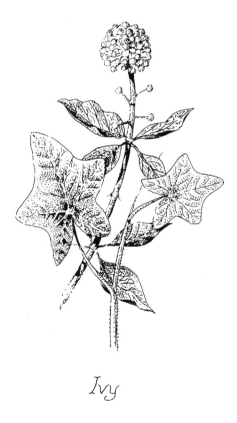

Ivy

J

A good wife and health are a man's best wealth.

JALAP. The common name for the Mexican plant *Ipomoea Jalapa* and the dried and powdered root was once used as a powerful **purgative**. Adapting the word jalap we use the slang word Jalop to mean a dose of medicine.

JAUNDICE. The yellowing of the skin and the whites of the eyes due to the absorption of bile formed by the **liver**. It is a condition found in many illnesses including pernicious anaemia, gall stones, hepatitis and liver damage. It was once believed that a sudden mental shock would cause jaundice.

It was better to keep out of the hands of 18th and 19th century doctors if suffering from jaundice as the standard cure of the day was **blood-letting**, a **vomit** and swallowing raw eggs.

The jaundice following **ague** was treated by Dr Benjamin Allen of Braintree Essex in the early 18th century with a novel ingredient; a spoonful of powdered peacock's dung mixed with any bitter drink. Dung seemed to be a favourite remedy of this particular doctor. See also **tuberculosis**.

John Wesley in his *Primitive Physic*, perhaps encouraged by the colour, thought **celandine** leaves in the shoes would cure jaundice.

In Shropshire as a cure they drank **saffron** water, again perhaps because of the colour.

An 18th-century treatment included a pill made of Castile **soap** to be taken every morning. Two centuries later this pill had become refined in the home remedy books, as Venice soap mixed with a few drops of aniseed.

Country people used **decoctions** of **nettles** and **burdocks**. Those with money hastened to **Cheltenham** for a cure – anything rather than the peacock dung.

JOINTS. For unspecified painful joints John Wesley in his *Primitive*

Physic recommended: 'Collect earth worms, thoroughly dry them, then powder them, and eat the same.'

A warm **poultice** or **mustard** poultice. See also **salt**.

JULEP. A sweet drink sometimes made from herbs with medicinal properties. **Mint** tea julep was made as a refreshing restorative and an old Cumbria Women's Institute cookery book gave the recipe as: 1 pint of freshly made tea, strained and sweetened, add 6 crushed fresh mint leaves and the juice of an orange and a **lemon** and keep cool. Just before serving add half a pint of **ginger** ale.

JUNIPER. *Juniperus communis*. An evergreen shrub commonly found on lime-rich heaths and moors of the north. In areas where juniper bushes grew country people made great use of them medicinally.

Berries were burnt on the fire to purify a house of infection, chewed to prevent **fever**, used in a **poultice** for **lumbago** and boiled to make a drink for digestive and urinary problems.

All this without knowing scientifically that the juniper berry has antiseptic properties, reduces **inflammation** and helps **digestion**. In addition juniper stimulates the uterus and juniper berries are used to flavour **gin** which may explain its many gynaecological uses in the past. See also **menses**.

According to folklore country people hung a flowering branch of juniper over the door in May to warn off witches. In the unlikely event of a dream involving juniper berries, this was seen as a sign of the birth of an heir or some other good fortune coming your way.

K

Better pay the cook than the doctor.

KAOLIN. Otherwise known as China clay. A smooth white powder of aluminium silicate used externally for skin irritations and internally for **diarrhoea**.

In the north a kaolin **poultice** was warmed in the oven and placed on the neck or chest to relieve the pain of meningitis and **pneumonia**.

Not everyone understood the hardening properties of kaolin once dried out. I was told the story of Uncle Jack of Sheffield who had pneumonia and came home to be nursed by his sister. When she had to pop out, another sister not medically minded, came round to keep an eye on him. She heated the kaolin and put it onto some

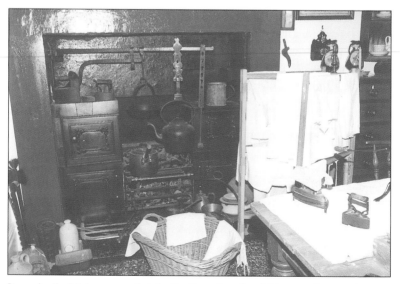

It was by the kitchen range that the family gathered and this was where mother cooked and made her home remedies. When anyone had a bad chest infection pans of water were boiled on the range and the kitchen filled with steam to help the patient breathe. (Photograph Ann Holubecki)

gauze but forgot to place a barrier of more gauze between the kaolin and Jack's very hairy chest. When the kaolin dried on his chest nothing would get it off and father had to get out the cut-throat razor and shave Uncle Jack's chest.

In hindsight an amusing story but also an example of how working class families looked after their own. Something has been lost from family life and few would consider now suffering any inconvenience to give a relation a bed and some nursing.

KIDNEY COMPLAINT. Another non-specific illness from the 1930s home remedy book for which a **decoction** of **marshmallow** root mixed with **lime** water and barley was recommended.

However if that did not work you were advised to drink an **infusion** of **comfrey** leaves. In the light of what we know now this was ill advised as this herb should not be taken internally.

See also **parsley**.

KINK COUGH. An old alternative name for **whooping cough**. The word 'kink' meant to hold the breath in spasms, from the Anglo Saxon 'cincian'.

KING'S EVIL. An old name for **scrofula**, the glandular form of **tuberculosis** in the lymph glands of the neck. From the 12th to the 18th century, in the days when royalty was esteemed as godlike, this condition was supposedly cured by the 'King's Touch' from the royal hand.

Charles I (1600–1649) even managed to go on curing after his death as it was believed that a cure could be had from a handkerchief dipped in his blood after his execution.

People paid large sums of money to travel, what must have seemed great distances, for the 'Touch'. Charles II (1630–1685) was particulary active in this form of healing, touching over 92,000 of his scrofulous subjects. All were given a 'touchpiece' of a gold angel which might explain the popularity of the remedy.

Queen Anne (1665–1714) was the last to carry out this task in England. The custom held on a little longer in Scotland as the

Young Pretender Bonnie Prince Charlie, unable to win back Scotland in 1745, had a go at touching some Scots – pretending to the last.

KOMPO. A renowned northern patent cough medicine first made in Leeds by J. F. White Ltd in 1885 and on sale until 1992. Sold under the name Dr White's Kompo it contained alcohol, capsicum, **cinnamon**, **cloves** and salicylic acid. I have known people who travelled the world with a bottle of this tucked in their luggage in case of emergencies; it is greatly missed.

L

Keep the blood pure and spare the leech.

LADY'S SLIPPER. *Cypripedium calceolus*. A native orchid, now very rare, found in woods on limestone in Yorkshire and County Durham. It was once regarded as a safe substitute for **opium** and the rhizomes were dried and used for **infusions**. It has sedative properties and was used in cases of **hysteria** and generally for anyone over excited.

LARYNGITIS. The inflammation of the larynx was soothed by a mixture of 1 tablespoon each of **honey**, glycerine, **lemon** juice or **vinegar**. An elderly lady told me this remedy worked when antibiotics failed.

LAUDANUM. Also known as Black Drop. This was **opium** dissolved in alcohol, a highly addictive and favoured narcotic of the upper classes in the 18th and 19th centuries, Writers and artists were most susceptible to the drug's effects of intense thoughts and wild creative ideas, all too soon followed by sleep. Increased doses of laudanum were needed as tolerance of the drug grew and someone on a high dose could take up to 400 drops a day. Many chemists made up their own brand of laudanum for the working poor who used it to dull the aches of **malaria** and **rheumatism**.

LAVENDER. *Lavandula angustifolia*, English lavender. An indispensable plant both in the garden and as an oil in the medicine cupboard. It is a natural antiseptic, antibiotic, and anti-depressant with healing, sedative and de-toxifying properties.

In the early Middle Ages lavender was used to sweeten linen and deter insects. It was scattered on the floors of houses and churches to protect against witchcraft. Lavender was grown in every monastic 'physik garden'.

The ancient Egyptians, Greeks and Romans used it extensively but we have overlooked its healing properties until recently, concentrating more on its use in disguising nasty smells.

LAXATIVE. See **aperient**.

LEAD POISONING. Lead ore (*galena*) has caused nothing but health problems. Lead poisoning causes dizziness, headaches, sickness ('lead colic'), anaemia, paralysis and death. The lead miners of the northern Pennines suffered unimaginable hardships: their life expectancy was 47. The lucky ones were those who left the remoteness of their villages and emigrated to America.

Lead mining also took place in the Mendips in Somerset where there were frequent conflicts between the farmers and miners. The lead smelting process was particulary harmful as the smoke, heavy with lead vapour, poisoned the vegetation, farm animals, water and fish in the streams.

The great age of lead mining in Britain coincided with the growth of manufacturing industries in the 18th and 19th centuries. The working conditions in the lead mines were appalling. Poor ventilation meant little oxygen, the miners worked with wet feet from the icy water draining from the mine workings and accidents were an everyday hazard. **Choke damp** caused by high levels of carbon dioxide left the miners with terrible headaches and gasping for breath. Working in this dust filled atmosphere the miners succumbed to 'the black spit', black mucous coughed up from the lungs and a sure sign that disability and death were soon to follow.

William Ewart, a surgeon to the London Lead Company, gave evidence at a public enquiry into the lead mining industry in 1862, 'I cannot call to mind having met with a miner who is not more or less affected with shortness of breathing before he is 40 years of age.'

So many manufacturing processes exposed other workers to lead poisoning: painters, plumbers, printers, glassmakers and especially pottery workers, where lead was used in the glaze. Possible lead poisoning was everywhere: lead water pipes meant contamination of the drinking water, household paint contained high levels of lead, the first food canning processes used lead to solder the tin, West Country cider made from apples crushed in a lead press caused lead poisoning called 'Devonshire colic'. It was even known for bakers to put white lead into their loaves to make a whiter bread! Many of the illnesses suffered over the last three centuries will have been because of lead poisoning.

LEAD POWDER. For centuries the English epitome of beauty was a pale white, unblemished skin. Queen Elizabeth 1 took the idea to extreme by using white lead powder as a face powder. Fashionable society for the next two centuries followed suit with powder and rouge made from lead generously applied to try and hide the **smallpox** scars.

Those making the white lead powder suffered the same symptons as the lead miners but with the additional burden of blindness before death. No one seems to have associated the illnesses with the lead or to have doubted that putting it onto the face was a good idea.

Lead poisoning was understood by the medical profession by the early 1900s. The *British Medical Journal* reported in 1905 that women in towns were making homemade lead pills to cause an abortion of an unwanted baby.

LEAMINGTON SPA. Once a small Warwickshire village of thatched cottages. The curative properties of Leamington's spring waters were known to the locals, who according to one historian used the saline spring for seasoning their meat! Unfortunately for those who could see the money being made in **Bath** and **Cheltenham**, from 'taking the waters', the first spring could not be developed commercially because it was on land owned by the Earl of Aylesford. He altruistically insisted the spring water be available free of charge to the poor of the parish.

It was not until two budding entrepreneurs, the local cobbler and the inn keeper Willam Abbotts, found a second saline spring on Abbotts' land that Leamington as a **spa** town could begin to flourish. Abbotts' Original Baths opened in 1786 and with the discovery of more saline and sulphurous springs, a splendid new Pump Room and Baths in 1814.

A fine new town was built between 1810 and 1840 with sweeps of terraces, crescents and elegant hotels. The 'Royal' prefix was graciously added to Leamington Spa during a visit by Queen

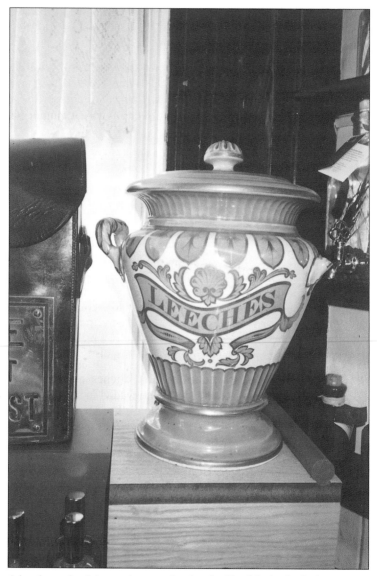

A handsome leech jar used to store leeches for blood-letting by barber surgeons, apothecaries and the local 'chymist'. It was a very popular treatment and was believed to relieve any 'congestion'. (By kind permission of John Farrah, Harrogate Toffee)

Victoria in 1838. European and British royalty, the aristocracy, politicians and celebrities all flocked there to bathe and drink the waters.

The spa treatment claimed to relieve the effects of **gout** and **rheumatism** and an **aperient** and some **blood-letting** were advised beforehand, to achieve maximum benefits from the waters. As the water had a laxative effect anyway it cannot have been an altogether pleasant experience.

The coming of the railways in the 1850s meant a decline for Leamington Spa as a fashionable watering place. High society could more readily travel by train to the coast for the latest new craze of **sea bathing**.

LEECH. A parasite that feeds off animals and humans by sucking blood. A physician in the Middle Ages was called a 'leech', reflecting the extensive use made of them as a 'cure' for most illnesses. This was to continue for centuries but blood sucking reached the height of its popularity in the 19th century. Leeches were applied to the 'congested' area to reduce the acute inflammation of vital organs. A leech bite keeps the blood flowing because of a substance in their saliva which stops blood clotting. Even today leeches can be used in micro-surgery.

LEECH GATHERING. Leeches inhabit ditches and ponds and were caught by bare-legged women who waded in and the leeches attached themselves to their feet and legs. The leeches were then transferred to a small barrel or keg suspended from the woman's waist. They suffered, as can be imagined, from a surfeit of leech bites and a broth made from tripe was applied to soothe and heal the bites. I can think of few more disagreeable jobs.

LEGS. **Ulcers** or **sores** on the legs were a common problem among the poor and the elderly. Poor nutrition and chronic ill health meant a weakened body unable to heal a wound or an infection. The following three remedies have all been used within living memory, very successfully, according to my informants.

The liquid left from soaking **bran** in water was used for bathing and healed a varicose ulcer.

An elderly farmer recommended **dock** leaves, shredded and boiled in a little water and the ulcer bathed in the liquid.

In Leicestershire pure **honey** was used on an ulcerated leg or a festering wound.

In earlier times John Wesley in his *Primitive Physic* advised washing the sore with brandy and applying **elder** leaves: 'This will dry up all the sores, though the leg were like an Honey-comb.'

LEMON. Rich in vitamin C both the juice and the rind were used in home treatments of **colds**. Lemons were not available all the year round and preserving them in buttermilk was recommended. It was known that lemon and **lime** juice helped to prevent **scurvy**. See also **heartburn**.

The Yorkshire farmer Edward Brown of Wensleydale was a great believer in the efficacy of a lemon and recorded in his commonplace book dated 1895:

'For the **liver** – Half the juice of a Lemmon [sic] in half a glass of water Night and Morning is good.'

'Unrivalled for relieving a **cough** – Equal parts of Lemon juice, glycerine and Brandy, dose half a teaspoonfull when necessary.'

A simple popular remedy in the early 1900s for **rheumatism** recommended boiling 2 lemons in 2 pints of water until reduced to a pint, then adding 2 ounces of **Epsom salts** and a large spoonful of **ginger**. You were advised to drink a wineglass a day – in other words an **aperient**!

See also **heartburn**.

LEPROSY. In the Middle Ages sickness was seen as a punishment for sin. Those who suffered from leprosy therefore suffered a double blow; not only were they shunned and kept in leper houses and asylums outside the town walls but it was seen as all their own fault.

Leprosy is a chronic disease caused by bacteria that attacks the skin and nerves. It was at its worse from the year 1000 to 1400 and untreated it led to hideous skin and body deformities with the loss of fingers and toes, paralysis and blindness. It was widely feared and contact with those affected was avoided at all costs. The leper was unable to work and forced to beg for alms from a not very sympathetic population, ringing a bell to announce his approach, swathed in garments to avoid his physical deformities giving offence.

Drinking the juice of a **houseleek** and a **decoction** from the inner bark of the English elm was thought to soothe the skin in leprosy but how likely was it that many lepers could lay their hands on these items? They therefore remained condemned and isolated.

LETHARGY. Believed to be almost always caused by **constipation**. However, an alternative to the inevitable **aperients** and **purgatives** was sniffing **vinegar** or **horseradish** up the nose.

LEUCORRHOEA. See **whites**.

LIME. Calcium oxide obtained by burning limestone. A solution was used as a disinfectant, and a wet sheet, soaked with lime water, was hung in the doorway of a sick room or draped around the bed to prevent infection spreading. It was also taken internally to settle the **bowels** and to help in **stomach disorders**. See also **bad legs**.

John Wesley in his *Primitive Physic* instructed: 'Lime-Water is made thus:- Infuse a pound of good quick lime, in 6 quarts of Spring water for 24 hours, decant and keep it for use.'

It was believed that lime wash painted on walls kept illness away. It was considered a great leap forward in the 1920s when the squalid huts that provided temporary living accommodation for Londoners down for the hop picking in Kent were lime-washed before occupation.

LIME JUICE. Fresh lime juice is very high in vitamin C and when issued to the British Navy from 1795 did away with **scurvy** overnight.

For small babies or the elderly suffering from a lack of appetite or no **teeth**, bread soaked in milk together with plenty of lime juice added to water was thought enough to keep them healthy.

LINIMENT. Another word for **embrocation** but usually made with oil. Every family had a favourite homemade liniment or rubbing oil for **lumbago, arthritis, muscular aches** and **rheumatism**.

One was: 2 ounces each of **turpentine**, spirits of **hartshorn, linseed** oil and **olive oil** mixed and shaken well.

A good liniment for arthritic joints was a mixture of **arnica, opodeldoc** and **olive oil**.

LINSEED. Seed from the common flax plant. Linseed meal was used as a **poultice** for a **boil** or a **carbuncle**. Linseed oil was used as a base for a **liniment**. See also **cough medicines**.

LIQUID PARAFFIN. Very popular at one time as a lubricant for those suffering from habitual **constipation**.

LIQUORICE. Also known as Spanish juice and used as an additional ingredient in a homemade **cough** or **cold** remedy and as a **laxative**. Liquorice does have medicinal properties and is said to be helpful to those suffering stomach **ulcers**. The Romans recognised that chewing the liquorice root gave them added vigour and in certain cases acted as an **aphrodisiac**. Bring on the Liquorice Allsorts!

The liquorice plant was grown around Pontefract from medieval times in the old West Riding of Yorkshire. The area became renowned for liquorice sold as Pomfret cakes. It was in 1760 that a local chemist George Dunhill added sugar and started making liquorice as sweets.

During the Second World War, when sweets were rationed, children bought liquorice roots from the chemist and chewed them as an alternative to sweets.

LIVER. A complex organ. The *Collins English Dictionary* defines the function of the liver as: 'It secretes bile, stores glycogen, detoxifies certain poisons, and plays an important part in the metabolism of carbohydrates, proteins and fats, helping to maintain a correct balance of nutrients.'

Not surprising that in the past many unspecified illnesses and a general feeling of being 'under the weather' were diagnosed as a problem with the liver. Even today we talk of feeling 'liverish'.

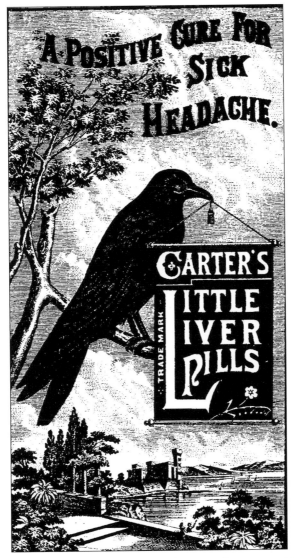

Until quite recently the liver was still seen as the cause of most unspecified illnesses so it was useful to have the word 'liver' in the name of your patent medicine. Carter's Little Liver Pills would have had minimal effect on the function of your liver but would have been excellent as a laxative. (By kind permission of the Thackray Museum, Leeds)

A 1930s home remedy book reflected this with several entries:

'Liver disease: Take of boiled milk 1 pint, very sharp syrup of **vinegar** 3 ounces, mix them, and after a little boiling, drink in the morning and walk upon it; continue for some days. This will cure a diseased liver.'

'Liver complaint: Thousands suffer from this complaint. Use this:- Boil gently a quarter of a pound of **brimstone** in a quart of water, when cold bottle it, and take a wineglassful twice a day. Those subject to this complaint could have no better remedy. Another active remedy is **dandelion** coffee, simply made from the dry root, roasted and ground, and used the same as coffee.'

'Liver enlarged: The diet should be of the simplest; drink nothing very hot and make free use of stewed **prunes** for a fortnight.'

'Liver sluggish: Equal parts of **hop** and **dandelion** tea . . . or **agrimony**, freely used as tea, strengthens a sluggish liver.'

Anything with a **lemon** in it was regarded as good for the liver. See also **asparagus**.

LIVERWORT. *Hepatica noblis*. An **infusion** of this toxic plant was recommended by **Culpepper**, who was still working from the **Doctrine of Signatures**, for diseases of the liver and kidneys. See also **mad dog bite**.

LOBELIA INFLATA. Also known as Indian tobacco and pukeweed. A powerful plant and harmful if eaten but much valued by those who followed **medical botany**. It has emetic and expectorant properties and increases perspiration. An **infusion** was once used in the treatment of **tuberculosis**.

LONG LIFE. *The Family Physician* of 1794 by Maximilian Hazlemore offered advice on how to 'Infallibly Prolong Life'. 'All who value health ought to be contented with eating one meal of flesh in the 24 hours and this ought to consist of one kind only. Do not drink **tea** in the morning. Take regular meals.'

LOW DIET. The early Victorians were great believers in the 'low diet' when feeling poorly. In order for the body to overcome sickness the stomach must not be 'overloaded'. It was a miserable diet which recommended:

'Breakfast – A pint of Panada [a mixture of flour and water], Water-gruel, or Milk-Pottage.
'Dinner Sunday and Thursday – A Pint of Broth, Two Ounces of Veal, or Four Ounces of Roots.'
For dinner on other days you could have 'a pint of Rice-Milk or a pint of Broth and Roots'.
You would indeed have been brought 'low' if you followed this regime for long.

LUMBAGO. A severe pain in the lumbar region of the back brought on by heavy work and muscle strain. In the past people were often susceptible to this through working in damp and cold conditions. Avoiding draughts and damp was a major consideration for the middle class. For example holidays were only be taken in hotels that actively promoted their 'Well-aired beds'. Older people never ventured out until 'the streets were aired'.

Warmth was everything and an extra layer of red **flannel** on the painful area was wrapped round your middle, under the vest, or a bandage dusted with **flowers of sulphur**.

Coal miners wore a piece of blanket over the top of a layer of Thermogene to help with lumbago right up to the 1950s.

Other manual workers after a hard day had someone iron their back with a flat iron, heated in front of the kitchen range. Leaning over the kitchen table, stripped to the waist, a layer of **brown paper** was laid on the back and the hot iron rubbed over the paper. I have been told that the warmth and pressure penetrating the lumbar region was quite blissful. See also **backache**.

For some having a potato in the pocket was enough to cure lumbago. To make sure you never suffered again you carried a potato in your pocket until it became completely shrivelled. I should imagine that at some point it had to be thrown away in the interests of congenial family life!

LUNGS. See **asthma**, **cough medicines**, **tuberculosis**.

M

The best physic is fresh air; the best pill plain fare.

MAD DOG BITE. People were haunted by the fear of being bitten by a mad dog. This was quite understandable given the fatal and horrific effects of rabies on humans before the French Professor of Chemistry Louis Pasteur developed a vaccine for it in 1885.

Opinion had it that the danger was less if you were bitten on the leg, rather than on any other part of the body – some comfort. Wet **salt** and soda were applied immediately.

Doctor Benjamin Allen of Braintree in Essex advised a curious form of nourishment in the 1700s if you were bitten. Kill the dog, cut out its liver, cook it and eat it. Perhaps an unusual form of revenge?

The Family Physician in 1794 published a lengthy cure. Dr Mead made great claims for 'he never knew this remedy to fail, although it has been tried in a thousand instances.' The good doctor's truthfulness may be called into question but judge for yourself.

'Take half an ounce of ash coloured ground **liverwort**, cleaned, dried and powdered, quarter of an ounce of black pepper. Mix these well together, and divide the powder into 4 doses, one of which must be taken every morning for 4 mornings successively, in half a pint of cow's milk, warm. After these 4 doses are taken, the patient must go into a **cold bath**, or cold spring or river, every morning for a month; he must be dipped all over, but not stay in with his head above water longer than half a minute, if the water be very cold. After this, he must go in 3 times a week for a fortnight longer. The person must be bled before he begins to use the medicine.'

Given that one of the symptoms of rabies is hydrophobia – fear of water – all this bathing was unlikely to help.

MADONNA LILY. *Lilium candidum*. The bulb and flowers were once used extensively for its healing and astringent properties. In the country areas of Wiltshire **cuts** and **bruises** were treated by applying a solution made from soaking the white petals in brandy.

MALARIA. See also **ague** and **quinine**. A fever transmitted by the bite of certain mosquitoes. From the 16th to the 19th century malaria was found in the Fens, parts of Essex, the Thames Estuary, North Kent, Romney Marsh, Yorkshire and the Somerset Levels.

It was a major cause of death and ill health. People were very aware of the danger, 17th century Essex clergymen refused to live on the Dengie Peninsula because of malaria, preferring the safety of Maldon. To prevent malaria you were advised to smoke to keep the mosquitoes at bay. Vast quantities of **opium** and **laudanum** were consumed, especially in the Fens, to deal with the unpleasant symptoms.

There were three stages in an attack first the feeling of extreme cold, then the opposite, extreme heat with pain throughout the body and then excessive sweating. Those who suffered from recurrent attacks of malaria became anaemic and weakened with a yellow tinge to the skin and an enlarged **liver** and spleen. For those suffering from malaria who could afford it, or those returning from the colonies, **Cheltenham** was the place to go to try for a cure.

Better hygiene, people no longer sharing living quarters with their animals, together with land drainage probably killed off malaria in this country. However we are warned that if our climate continues to get warmer, we could see the return of a lesser form of malaria – *plasmodium vivax*.

MALVERN. In 1756 a Dr Wall extolled the medicinal virtues of the waters of Malvern Wells because of their purity:

'The Malvern Water, says Dr. John Wall,
Is famous for containing just nothing at all.'

This made Malvern water very different from other **spa** waters with their saline, chalybeate or **sulphur** content and Great Malvern quickly grew, from a small Worcestershire village, to a popular **spa** town with all the hotels and lodgings needed for the medical tourist trade.

In 1842 Doctors Wilson and Gully brought hydrotherapy – the Water Cure – from Austria. Dr Wilson's speciality was the dawn **wet sheet** cure, followed by a brisk walk in the hills to drink fresh spring water – all this before breakfast, which was usually **oatmeal** porridge. **Tea** drinking was banned.

For those used to rich foods, alcohol and society life this healthy regime of bathing, fresh air, water, simple food and early bed must have done them a power of good: that it was also expensive meant it was all the more successful.

MARGATE. The oldest and most famous resort in Kent. In 1791 Dr John Coakley Lettson founded 'The Margate Infirmary for the relief of the Poor whose Diseases require Seabathing', to become famous countrywide with the shorter name, The Royal Sea Bathing Hospital. It was here that people came to be treated for **scrofula** and **tuberculosis**.

A Quaker, Benjamin Beale, originally a Glover and Breeches maker, was upset by the sights of those indulging in the new **seabathing** craze. He devised a bathing machine with a modesty hood in 1753, where you could splash around, in what was virtually your own, private bathing pool measuring 13ft × 18ft.

Following the popular advice of the day from Dr Richard Russell **sea water** was also drunk, unfortunately taken from the sea at Margate only 50 yards from the sewer. These treatments were all kill or cure.

MARIGIOLD. *Calendula officinalis.* The common or pot marigold. Long known as a medicinal herb for its healing and soothing properties. Grown in gardens since the Middle Ages it was once used extensively on **wounds, sores, ulcers** and **warts** and to soothe **inflammation**. The petals were said to aid digestion and used to colour food.

The 1930s home remedy book believed in the virtues of the marigold: 'Of great value for **palpitations**, **hysteria**, female obstructions, **measles** and **ulcers**; it will heal any sore or wound quickly; use inwardly or outwardly. Marigold tea comforts the heart exceedingly.' See also **bubonic plague**.

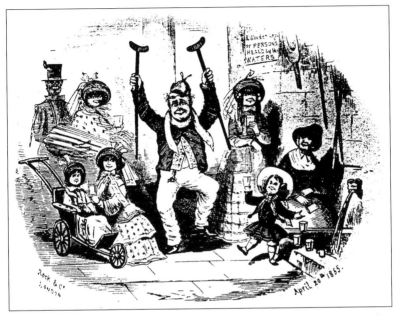

An 1885 claim for what Malvern waters could do for you. The notice on the wall advises that hanging there are the 'Crutches and Wooden Legs of Persons heal'd by the Waters.' Perhaps not completely truthful! (Reproduced by kind permission of Worcestershire County Council Cultural Services)

MARSHMALLOW. *Althaea officinalis*. All parts of this plant have medicinal properties and are said to soften and heal. The root can be boiled and eaten as a rather unlikely vegetable and a **decoction** of the root once formed part of a remedy for a **kidney complaint**. See also **housemaid's knee**.

MEADOWSWEET. *Filipendula ulmaria*. Also called Queen of the Meadows. Used since ancient times as a 'strewing herb' scattered on floors to disguise smells. The plant contains salicylic acid, first discovered in 1839, from which aspirin is derived. An older name was *Spiraea ulmaria* and it was from this we get the word aspirin.

Tea made from meadowsweet was said to cheer up those pining or thwarted in love but at the same time you had to eat (female) biscuits made from **nettles** and (male) biscuits made from **dandelion**.

MEASLES. Before immunisation measles was a serious, highly infectious disease and there were many epidemics. As well as a rash the eyes became sore and red and the sick child was kept in a darkened room, often with a blue sugar bag over the light bulb to subdue the light.

A 1920s home remedy book advised 'the free use of **lemon** or **saffron** water sweetened to taste.' See also **ivy** and **cleavers**.

In 18th century Shropshire they used a cure similar to the one for **whooping cough** but instead of a donkey the child was passed over and under a dancing bear!

MEDICAL BOTANY. The unfortunately named Albert I. Coffin brought Medical Botany to Britain in 1838 from America. It was part of a wave of alternative medicines which were critical of the prescribing methods of doctors, with their **heroic** doses and heavy use of **laudanum, blood-letting** and **purging**. The medical profession in turn was pretty 'sniffy' about Coffin.

He set up his 'Botanic Colleges' all over the North and Midlands and his ideas found favour amongst the working class, Nonconformists and other members of the 'awkward squad' who refused to accept that conventional doctors necessarily knew best.

Medical Botany was based on the theory that disease was caused by cold in the body. It used plant drugs mainly *lobelia inflata* and **cayenne** to produce great internal heat to force out the cold.

MEDICINAL JAM. This 1930s recipe from Northumberland is an **aperient** masquerading as a teatime treat:

Take a pound each of raisins and prunes and remove stones from prunes. Finely chop prunes, raisins and a quarter of a pound of blanched almonds. Leave to soak overnight in 1 pint of water. Next day add a pound of Demerara sugar, bring to the boil and cook for 30 minutes. Pour into hot jars and seal immediately – delicious on brown bread.

MEDICINES. Many ordinary people had an uncomplicated view of disease and kept their medicines simple. Self-help and prescribing were a virtue and the following are examples of how you kept your family out of the doctor's hands:

A Leicestershire gentleman, according to his granddaughter, had three bottles as his medicine chest:

White oil – horse embrocation to ease stiff joints.
Black oil – molasses and **linseed oil** for internal ills.
Green oil – **lemon** juice and cider **vinegar** for colds and chest infections.

A Yorkshire childhood recalled by a lady from Sheffield remembered three brown earthenware stewpots on the top of the kitchen range:

The first – scalded **lemons** with **Epsom salts** to clear the blood.
The second – **senna** pods for a laxative.
The third – stewed barley and the liquid from this was drunk to clear your 'waterworks'.

From my Cumbrian childhood, a friend's mother had refined this even further, she believed that you only needed two items:

Milk of Magnesia and Syrup of Figs.

MELANCHOLY. A 1930s home remedy book advised drinking a tea made of equal parts of **agrimony** and **rosemary**. See also **cold baths** and **wormwood**.

MENOPAUSE. See **change of life** and **sarsaparilla**.

MENSES. The Interruption of the Menses, as it was so delicately called, referred to a painful or late menstruation or 'period'.

To 'bring down the courses' meant to start a period and if you were irregular it was seen as 'a loss of vital power'.

John Wesley in his *Primitive Physic* had advice on the subject and thought a spoonful morning and evening of 'juice of Syrup of Brooklime' – a kind of speedwell to be found in ditches – would do the trick.

The Family Physician of 1794 can only have been writing for young ladies of good family and fortune when it advised on 'Obstructions in Young Girls'. Few of the working class could afford the time or the money to follow these very sympathetic instructions:

'If her health and spirits begin to decline place her in a situation where she can enjoy the benefit of fresh air and agreeable company. Then let her eat wholesome food, take sufficient exercise and amuse herself in the most agreeable manner and Nature will do her proper work. . . Females ought to be exceedingly cautious of what they eat and drink at the time they are out of order. [Avoid] Everything that is cold, or apt to sour on the stomach such as fruit, butter, milk, fish. Filings of iron may be infused in wine for two to three weeks and [take] half a wineglass a day.'

Dr Thomas Graham in his *On the Diseases of Females* 1841 thought the air and water of **Tunbridge Wells** an ideal place to go for 'retention of the menses' but more importantly, 'Most patients will be comforted and benefited by wearing flannel drawers in the autumn and winter.'

'Dr' Coffin in his **medical botany** recommended **juniper** berries to 'promote monthly terms' and his assistant John Skelton advised that washing with **vinegar** and water once a week would help.

In more recent times women in the towns used the sterilised outer bark of **slippery elm** if the monthly period was late, inserting it into the vagina and leaving it there for about 45 minutes.

The herb **pennyroyal**, drunk like tea, was known by countless countrywomen to bring on a monthly period.

Every woman over a certain age can remember someone, if not themselves, being treated very successfully with **gin** and hot water sweetened with sugar for a painful period. See also **southernwood**.

MENSTRUAL MYTHS. To read in the Bible, Leviticus 15 verses 19 to 24, helps to understand the horror with which this time of the month was regarded, especially by men: 'And if a woman have an issue, and her issue in her flesh be blood, she shall be put apart seven days: and whosoever toucheth her shall be unclean.' It goes on to say that everything she lies, sits and sleeps on is unclean and that if a man touch any of these he too is unclean and must immediately bathe. This can explain why in many religions men and women worship separately.

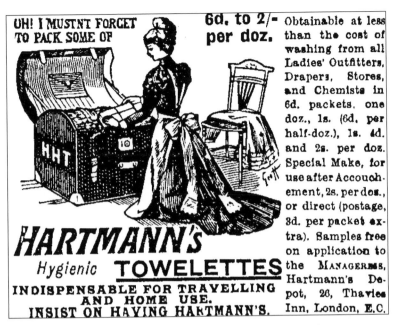

UH! I MUSTN'T FORGET TO PACK SOME OF

6d. to 2/- per doz.

Obtainable at less than the cost of washing from all Ladies' Outfitters, Drapers, Stores, and Chemists in 6d. packets, one doz., 1s. (6d. per half-doz.), 1s. 4d. and 2s. per doz. Special Make, for use after Accouchement, 2s. per doz., or direct (postage, 3d. per packet extra). Samples free on application to the MANAGERESS, Hartmann's Depot, 26, Thavies Inn, London, E.C.

HARTMANN'S *Hygienic* **TOWELETTES**

INDISPENSABLE FOR TRAVELLING AND HOME USE.
INSIST ON HAVING HARTMANN'S.

From *The Lady's World* of 1899. Sanitary towels or 'towlettes' as they were delicately known, were only for the better off. Poorer women had to make do with old rags and wash them for further use once soiled.

So with this background is it any wonder that the 'old wives tales' about the menstrual period should be rich and varied and that normal life practically ceased for a few days every month. Here are some I have collected but I am sure there will be others I have missed:

Do not wash your hair, have a bath or go swimming or you will catch a cold.
Do not play any sport as it will make you weak.
Do not ride a bicycle.
Do not eat ice cream. See **menses** for the advice from 1794.
Do not sit on anything cold or put your feet in cold water or the menstrual blood will rush to your head and send you mad.
Do not have a perm – there is some truth in this – as the perm does not 'take'.
Do not handle raw meat, especially a cured ham as it will become rancid.

Do not go into the dairy or the milk will go off and do not on any account attempt to make butter or cheese. An old 17th century belief, very much along the same lines, thought a menstruating woman could turn the wine rancid and the sugar black.

Lastly a myth peculiar to Lincolnshire, do not walk in the countryside or you will attract snakes!

MIGRAINE. Sometimes written as megrim or megraine and an altogether more intense and debilitating affliction than a **headache**.

The Lady's World of 1898, whose readership one might suppose suffered from migraines, offered the advice:

'Cod liver oil – a teaspoonful once daily after breakfast and then gradually increase the dose to a tablespoonful. The bodily and nervous systems should be braced up by means of good food and tonics. Many sufferers derive the geatest possible benefit by prolonging their rest in bed till 11 am. Apply a hot water bottle to the feet. If instead of disturbance of vision preceding the headache there is a feeling of depression, 20 drops of tincture of **henbane** with same quantity of spirit of chloroform will soothe the nervous system. If the headache is only slight a cup of coffee followed by a drive will soon get rid of it.'

That a poisonous plant like **henbane** could be used to treat a migraine may well explain why many upper class women suffered so much chronic sickness.

An altogether simpler idea to cure a migraine was sipping a glassful of very cold water slowly. This remedy was unlikely to appeal to those who needed a cure to be complicated for it to work.

MINT. *Mentha*. There are at least thirty different species of mint. In the Middle Ages mint was used as a 'strewing herb' to disguise the smells. Hanging a bunch of mint in the doorway was thought to deter flies. In the 17th century it was believed that sniffing mint 'strengthens the brain, and preserves the Memory'.

As an **infusion** it aids digestion, which is why mint sauce is eaten with lamb. It can also calm **flatulence**.

A thimbleful of mint and **witch hazel** was said to be very good for lifting the spirits. See also **julep**.

MISTLETOE. *Viscum album*. A highly toxic plant shrouded in mystery and superstition and long associated with the Druids. If we think about mistletoe at all now it is only as a Christmas custom, copied from the Scandinavians, of hanging it in the house where if we are lucky we might get a kiss under it.

The leaves and stems of mistletoe were used medicinally right up to the 1930s as the sedative properties were said to help those suffering from **St Vitus's Dance**. An interesting mix of superstition and Christianity believed that mistletoe placed on a church altar on Christmas Eve was especially potent medically.

MORNING SICKNESS. An elderly lady told me that the quickest way to cure morning sickness in her day was to use an outdoor privy! Others recommended that nothing should be eaten after 6 pm.

In Wiltshire any **infusion** of **mint** or **golden rod** was drunk to relieve the sickness.

MORTIFICATION. Another name for gangrene. When I was researching a previous book I was shown a fascinating **commonplace book** from the early 1800s, once belonging to a Shipley cobbler. Besides mending shoes he did a bit of illegal money lending on the side and his book was a mixture of mysterious accounts, a recipe for invisible ink and some medical notes. 'Apply a poultice of flour, **honey** and water with a little **yeast** to stop a mortification.'

On similar lines a 1930s home remedy book advised making a poultice of flour, **marshmallow** water, brown sugar and **yeast**.

A more bizarre idea from a 1920s home remedy book suggested dusting the mortification with fine sugar.

MOTHER SEIGEL. Mother Seigel's Syrup and Mother Seigel's Operating Pills were popular patent remedies readily available in the 1900s. All the home remedy books until the 1940s gave the ingredients for you to either make your own or ask the chemist to make them for you. The syrup and pills contained, among other

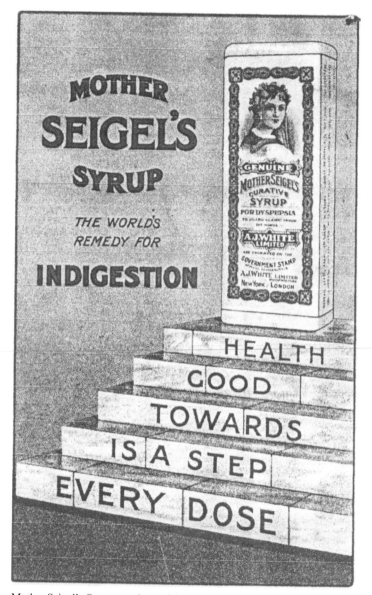

Mother Seigel's Syrup may have claimed to be a remedy for indigestion but it contained powerful laxative ingredients: aloes, borax, gentian, capsicum, liquorice and treacle. (By kind permission of the Thackray Museum, Leeds)

things, three powerful **purgatives**, especially in the doses recommended: **liquorice**, scammony (an Asian convolvulus plant), and bitter **aloes**. However, taken to excess the powerful purging action acted as an **abortificant** and desperate women used it as such.

Who was Mother Seigel? In all probability she did not exist. Originally an American product the company, along with many others in the early 1900s, gave their medicines names that would link them in the public mind with the Shakers or Quakers. These were honest, God fearing folk with a reputation for thrift, temperance and knowledge of herbs. You were surely able to trust any medicine coming from such a respectable source. Unfortunately it was just so much advertising 'spin'.

In this country Mother Seigel's medicines were manufactured by A.J. White who advertised them as 'A remedy for the habitual costiveness from which women frequently suffer, and for all the distressing symptoms peculiar to the season of change.'

MOUSE PIE. An unusual 19th century remedy cooked by mother and eaten by small boys who continually wet the bed. Or were they just threatented with it. . .?

See also **whooping cough**.

MUMPS. Once called 'The Branks'. Highly infectious with painful swelling of the face and **neck**. Urban myth had it that if a grown man caught mumps he would become sterile and fathers stayed well clear of a child's sickroom. There is some truth in this as in a few cases mumps may cause inflammation of the testicles resulting in atrophy – wasting away.

MUSCULAR ACHES. See **embrocation** and **liniment**.

MUSTARD. *Brassica nigra* – black mustard is stronger medicinally than *Sinapis alba* – white mustard. The pungent mustard seed has been used in home remedies for centuries. Mixed with water it becomes a volatile oil which is highly irritating to the skin.

Mustard is a powerful emetic as a teaspoonful of mustard in a glass of warm water can swiftly bring on vomiting. See also **vertigo**.

For warmth and to stimulate the circulation cold feet were soaked in a bowl of hot water and mustard.

Mustard was a favourite ingredient in many remedies for a **cold** and chesty **cough**.

A mustard **plaster** acted as a counter irritant to treat **rheumatism**, painful **joints** and congested **lungs**. The mustard could be mixed with water or **linseed oil** and applied to the skin but always making sure you had a piece of gauze, linen or brown paper between you and the mustard. However if you used egg white instead, the skin would not blister quite so much! See also **blister, to**.

MUTTON SUET. An unlikely medicine but people used this easily obtained commodity to treat **sores** and **chapped hands**. When melted it could be smeared onto a bandage and wrapped round a **cut** or bruise. See also **nappy rash**.

It was a brave person who could drink, and keep down, this old cure found in a family **commonplace book**: 'Finely shred 1 ounce of Mutton Suet, and allow to simmer in 1 pint of Milk for half an hour. Strain through muslin and drink while hot.

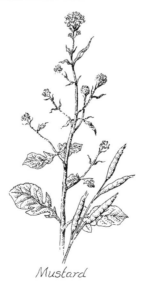

Mustard

N

NAPPY RASH. Once upon a time every mother had 2 dozen cotton nappies to see her through until a baby was 'dry'. For approximately 2 years, if you were lucky, these nappies had to be soaked in disinfectant then boiled and dried every day. I look with amazement at today's mothers and the disposable nappies and feel very old as I think, 'They don't know they're born.'

All the boiling and the quickly soggy droopy nappies meant there was a problem with chafing or a rash. To prevent a nappy rash mothers up to the 1950s were advised, after bathing the baby, to rub on the baby's bottom starch or cornflour.

To soothe a nappy rash the advice was to spread on **mutton suet** or the white of an egg.

NECK. John Wesley in his *Primitive Physic* recommended drinking half a pint of **sea water** every other day for swollen glands, such as those suffered in **mumps**.

If this could not be tolerated a gargle made from a **decoction** of **nettles** was a better option.

From a 1930s home remedy book for a swollen neck: 'Get the cheapest **gin** you can. Dip a handkerchief in it and sleep all night with this tied over the glands. In bad cases try painting with **iodine**.'

There was a widely held belief that wearing a coral necklace or one made of red beads would prevent swollen glands.

A stiff neck was relieved by spreading a mixture of **mustard** and **vaseline** onto a cloth and wearing it round the neck.

NEGUS. Named after Colonel Francis Negus who in the 18th century invented a sweetened drink of port, **lemon** and spices. Unlikely as it might seem this rather splendid drink was regarded as a treatment for **gout**.

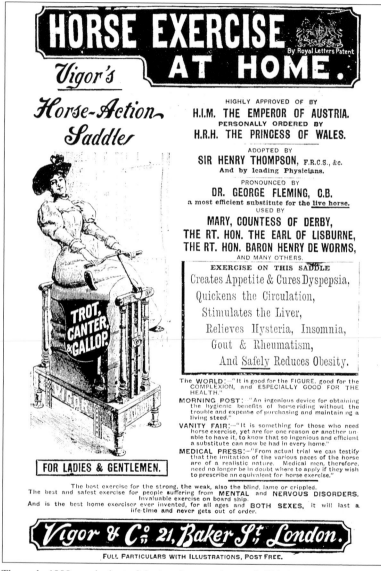

The early 1900s equivalent of the 'work out at the gym'. This horse exercise was recommended for the weak, the blind, lame or crippled and as the best and safest exercise for those suffering from mental and nervous disorders. The side saddle version looks positively dangerous! (Joe Pie Picture Library)

NERVOUS DISORDERS. A complex subject for which there are many symptoms and just as many causes. Put simply, it was quite acceptable for women of a certain class to show a delicacy of feeling that could easily topple over into debilitating nervousness and illness. Often boredom and the inability, because of social convention, to pursue interests outside family and home, prevented them from reaching their full potential. This left women with the only alternative of being interesting by being ill. There was an expression used to describe this type of woman, 'Pale and interesting'.

Sensitive men who perhaps had repressed homosexual thoughts, or who were required to work at jobs for which they had no enthusiasm or were unfitted, also fell prey to unspecified 'nerves'. Suffering from one's 'nerves' was not a preoccupation of the working class – they had other, more pressing concerns.

The term 'neurasthenia' was a popular one in Victorian society. It meant a condition of nervous physical and mental exhaustion for which no physical cause could be found. It is interesting to note that the heyday of the various **spa** towns coincided with the neurasthenic hypochondria of the affluent classes.

Even the no nonsense Yorkshire farmer Edward Brown of Wensleydale noted in his **commonplace book** of 1895: 'Citrate of Iron and **quinine**, for Tooth ache, Nerves & Making Blood – Nothing to equal it.'

Nervous people were recommended to drink a tea made from **sage** and **thyme** and not to drink **coffee** and very little **tea**. See also **female constitution**.

According to a 1930s home remedy book, nervous debility accompanied by **palpitations** 'is greatly relieved by mixing two drachms [a drachm was one eighth of a fluid ounce] each of chloric ether, **tincture** of gentian, **sal volatile**, iodide of potassium to each half pint of cold water (first boiled), take a tablespoonful 3 times a day. As a stimulant it has no equal.'

A more humdrum solution to help with your 'nerves' was to take up knitting!

NETTLES. *Urtica dioica* also known as stinging nettle. Without knowing the chemical constituents, of what we think of as a weed, people in the past recognised a good thing when they saw it. Fresh young nettles were picked enthusiastically and used in many home remedies and **spring tonics**. The nettle contains vitamins A and C, iron, formic acid, ammonia, silicic acid and histamine. It has astringent, tonic and toning properties, improves the circulation and purifies the system. All this from a weed!

Springtime meant spring cleaning in more senses than one; both the house and one's internal workings received attention. This was the time for a good **purge** and a clear out and for that purpose you picked the young nettle shoots and leaves.

In country areas you drank nettle water with extra **brimstone** and treacle to pep up sluggish **bowels** and to clear **spots**. You could also gargle with it for a **sore throat** or swollen **neck** and some lint soaked in nettle water and stuffed up the nose would stop a **nosebleed**.

Young nettles were cooked and served like spinach or made into a soup with onions, potatoes and chicken stock.

Homemade nettle beer was considered a very healthy drink.

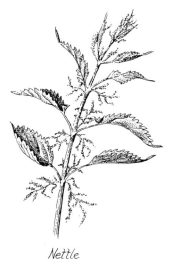

Nettle

Edna Simpson's Nettle Beer

Rinse, drain and boil 2lbs of young nettle tops for 15 minutes. Strain into a bowl and add the peel and juice (but not the zest) of 2 **lemons**, 1lb of demerara sugar and 1 ounce cream of tartar. Stir well and when cold add some **yeast**. Keep covered with a cloth in a warm room for 3 days then strain and bottle. Keep a week before drinking.

See also **overweight**.

A nettle sting could act as a counter-irritant to the pain of **rheumatism** and the Romans were said to love nothing more than a roll in a patch of nettles to overcome the aches of a cold English winter.

NETTLE RASH. See **dock leaf**, **parsley** and **stings**.

NEURALGIA. Pain in a sensory nerve often brought on by cold and damp. A cutting cold wind could bring on neuralgia in the face and the cure of **elderberry** and port wine was very comforting.

Relief was to be had from heat and to that end it was recommended to place **brimstone** in the sole of a sock but 'contrary to the pain side'.

Other forms of heat applied to the painful area were **cayenne** sprinkled onto a hot flannel or hot **hops** placed in a bag. 'Try it at once,' urged a 1930s home remedy book.

From the same book came the promise of a certain cure. ' A Lancashire gentleman paid 10 guineas for this prescription, and was well satisfied. Tincture of Gelsemium.' This was the powdered root of the yellow jasmine which was a sedative, although those taking it at the time would not have realised.

NIGHTMARE. To prevent a nightmare you were told never to eat cheese just before going to bed. A country superstition believed that you should always have the bed facing from the east to the west, never north to south.

However, if none of this worked a 1920s home remedy book advised you to drink an **infusion** of **thyme**.

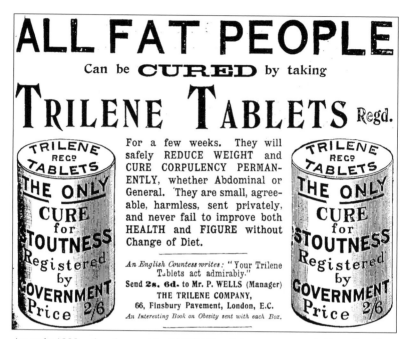

ALL FAT PEOPLE

Can be **CURED** by taking

TRILENE TABLETS Regd.

For a few weeks. They will safely REDUCE WEIGHT and CURE CORPULENCY PERMAN-ENTLY, whether Abdominal or General. They are small, agree-able, harmless, sent privately, and never fail to improve both HEALTH and FIGURE without Change of Diet.

An English Countess writes : " Your Trilene Tablets act admirably."

Send **2s. 6d.** to Mr. P. WELLS (Manager)
THE TRILENE COMPANY,
66, Finsbury Pavement, London, E.C.
An Interesting Book on Obesity sent with each Box.

TRILENE RECD TABLETS THE ONLY CURE for STOUTNESS Registered by GOVERNMENT Price 2/6

An early 1900s advertisement for 'All Fat People' was accompanied by a list of glowing testimonials. A lady from Liverpool wrote, 'I lost nearly a stone from taking one box.' A Liverpool gentleman wrote on behalf of his wife, 'Who was many years growing so stout . . . the Tablets soon reduced the same completely. You have our united thanks.' Impossible to know what they might have contained but probably a powerful purgative.

NITRE. A favourite in the medicine cabinet. Sometimes known as **saltpetre** or potassium nitrate. Sweet spirit of nitre was found in a favourite digestive tonic, **Indian brandee**. It settled the stomach and dilated the blood vessels, in some circumstances it caused sweating and acted as a diuretic. I was told of an elderly Leeds man who swore by nitre and took a drop in warm water if he was stopping in and a drop in cold water if he was going out. He was still digging his own garden when he died at 94.

NITS. The tiny parasitic head lice which live on the scalp and whose eggs are to be found attached to the hair. The school 'nit nurse', affectionately named 'Nitty Nora' at my old school, was once a regular visitor and it was seen as a great shame to be found having nits in the hair. The claim that nits only liked clean hair 'cut no ice' with mothers like mine, who forbade me to play with a girl she felt was responsible for my infestation.

Long hours were spent removing nits with the fine-toothed 'dickie' or 'biddy' comb. Other ways of getting rid of them included washing the hair in a mixture of paraffin and **olive oil** or rubbing on Geneva **gin, turpentine** and **quassia** chips.

NOSEBLEED. A cold key down the back was the favourite way to stop a nosebleed and was infinitely preferable to the old Northamptonshire folk cure of killing a toad with a sharp pointed instrument and hanging it in a bag round the neck. See also **nettles** and **yarrow**.

NOSTRUM. A **quack** or patent remedy. See **quacks**.

NUTMEG. *Myristica fragrans*. A bitter astringent herb once used as a tonic medicinally but now restricted to cooking. Adding grated nutmeg to a dish was believed to be an aid to digestion.

I know a lady of great distinction, who to this day, always has a nutmeg about her person to keep **rheumatism** at bay.

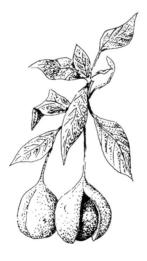

Nutmeg

O

Costiveness cannot exist long without danger to health.

OAK. The bark of an English oak is high in tannins and has astringent anti-inflammatory properties and for a long time was used in folk medicine.

A 1930s home remedy book recommended a **decoction** of oak bark to be used as a wash for **ulcers**, bleeding **piles** and a bloody **flux**.

OATMEAL. Oatmeal, especially eaten as porridge, was a cheap food for the poor. It undoubtedly was wholesome and filling and among its many virtues a 1920s home remedy book proclaimed, 'A pound of oatmeal gives a man as much strength as 3 pounds of lean beef, 3 pounds of boiled ham, 9 bottles of Bass's pale ale or 6 bottles of **Guinness**'s stout.'

It was a favourite ingredient for a hot **poultice** to relieve **earache** or draw a **boil**.

Current thinking and science tell us that oats are a good thing as they reduce high cholesterol levels and are high in *avena sativa* which is said to improve one's sexual energy. So, although it might not be very sexy, a bowl of porridge followed by some **liquorice** might be just the thing for a flagging libido.

See also **chapped hands, Malvern** and **post natal depression**.

OFFICINALIS. *Officina* is the Latin name for workshop. In the Middle Ages the officina was the storeroom in a monastery where the herbs were kept and made into medicines by the monks. From this the custom began of labelling any plant that had once been used medically as *officinalis*.

OINTMENT. An older name for a healing ointment was salve. A good housewife would have a go at making her own ointment, especially for **chapped hands**. The best ointment was made from cow's cream buried a day or two in a cloth in the garden.

An old fashioned **sulphur** salve for the skin, made easily at home,

mixed equal amounts of lard and **flowers of sulphur**. See also
pennywort.

An old superstition believed that no ointment should be put on
with the first finger as it was thought to contain 'poison'. Instead
the third finger should be used as it is harmless and in addtion said
to be a lucky finger.

OLIVE OIL. Recommended by Mrs Beeton in her 1861 *Book of
Household Management* as a cure for **flatulence**. It was not
regarded as having any role in cookery for it never occurred to
anyone to cook in anything other than animal fats. Its role was
firmly medicinal; a commodity to be bought from a chemist in
small bottles and used as a lubricant in homemade medicines. It
was most commonly used as a cure for **earache** and to soothe
stomach **ulcers**.

A drop of olive oil was useful for removing painful grit or a speck
from the eye.

A tablespoon a day was recommended for **indigestion**.

After the austerity and rationing of the war years the cookery
writer Elizabeth David introduced the British, in the 1950s, to the
flavours and colours of Mediterranean food. Olive oil was thus
released from the medicine cupboard.

ONION. The onion has long been used medicinally for its antiseptic
and expectorant properties. However, in early times hanging a
bunch of onions outside the door was thought to keep away the
plague and **cholera**. Times move on but the safe-guarding
properties lingered in folk memory and people still, until quite
recently, placed a cut onion on a saucer in a room wherever
anyone had been with a **cold**.

John Wesley in his *Primitive Physic* thought an onion would help
cure the **palsy**. 'Shred white Onions, and bake them gently in an
earthen pot, 'till they are soft. Spread a thick plaister of this, and
apply it to the be-numb'd parts.' See also **plaster**.

A **poultice** made with roasted onions was thought to have a good
effect on a **tumour**.

OPODELDOC. An old name for soap liniment and used as one of the ingredients in a rubbing oil or homemade **liniment**.

OPIUM. An addictive, narcotic drug extracted as a juice from the unripe seed of the opium poppy containing alkaloids such as morphine and codeine and therefore a good painkiller.

During the 1800s opium was widely used in any number of patent medicines from **teething** powders for babies to cough and cold medicines. In the West Midlands 'Godfrey's Cordial' was a very popular sedative or 'comforter' and contained opium and treacle.

Opium was used extensively in conventional medicine. The 1841 book, *On the Diseases of Females* by Dr Thomas Graham recommended it as of great value in severe menorrhagia.

Buying and selling opium-based products was part of everyday life and pills and potions were easily obtained from shops and markets. **Laudanum** was used extensively by those who could afford it, while 'poppy tea' made from the seeds was a cheaper alternative. Opium poppies were grown in England and although not as strong as the Indian poppy were used to treat the effects of **ague**. This explains why they were grown and used so much in the low-lying marshy Fens. There was high mortality from opium use in Lincolnshire and also a much higher rate of addiction and use of opium in the remote, undrained parts of Cambridgeshire, Huntingdonshire and Norfolk than in the rest of England.

Opium was also the reason why at one time the people of the Fens were thought a bit on the slow side as smoking the sap and drinking the tea meant they were all seriously 'out of it'. The men were called 'Fen Tigers' and said to be fierce when roused but small in stature and dark with a yellow tinge to their skin because of the jaundice caused by the **ague**.

The sale of opium went unregulated until the Pharmacy Act of 1868 and even then the rules were not strictly enforced. Many were unknowingly addicted to patent medicines, others were only just beginning to realise the dangers.

ORANGE PEEL. Not really a remedy or cure, but an interesting snippet of social history told me by a lady who remembered doing it. In County Durham the girls chewed a piece of orange peel before going to a dance because it made their eyes sparkle!

OYSTERS. Now a delicacy they were once the staple fare of Victorian England. They were considered, 'the unrivalled diet for brain workers, and offered strenuous opposition to the attack of the **influenza** fiend.' Once very popular as an **aphrodisiac** with good reason as they contain zinc which is needed to maintain the male libido. Eating Whitstable oysters was considered a cure for **dyspepsia**. See also **barrenness**.

OVERWEIGHT. Advice from a 1930s home remedy book: 'For stout persons to keep down burdensome fat, use a wine-glassful of the best Hollands **gin** 2 or 3 times a week, and avoid the use of much bacon or bread; or simply 20 to 30 crushed **nettle** seeds, taken night and morning daily will prevent burdensome fat surrounding the kidneys and stopping the heart. Tried with good results.' If only it were that simple!

P

Passion has a greater influence on health than people are aware of.

PALPITATIONS. This is when one becomes aware of the abnormal beating of the heart, often very rapidly. There are many causes, for example a sudden fright, feeling anxious, drinking too much **tea**, **coffee** and alcohol, **dyspepsia,** after strenuous exercise or occasionally, and more seriously, heart disease.

A 1930s home remedy book advised a no nonsense drink of cold water with a pinch of salt in it.

John Wesley in his *Primitive Physic* also recommended drinking cold water, sniffing **vinegar** and carrying a hare's foot in the pocket as this would prevent palpitations caused by heartburn.

PALSY. Another word for paralysis. See **sage** and **onions**.

Plunging the patient into a cold bath was thought to startle the afflicted into some movement followed by sweating and a good rub down.

PAREGORIC. Once bought from the chemist and used extensively in many homemade **cough medicines** and for an upset stomach. It was made up of **opium**, aniseed oil, **benzoic acid** and **camphor**.

The Wensleydale farmer Edward Brown in his **commonplace book** dated 1895 demonstrated the popularity of paregoric when it appeared twice on the same page. Firstly in a cough medicine containing an extra slug of **laudanum,** more aniseeds, **peppermint** and treacle and secondly as a stomach medicine with all the ingredients for a good **purge**, including **Turkey rhubarb**.

PARSLEY. *Petroselinum crispum* – the sort used in cooking and found in a pot by the kitchen door. The Greeks and Romans knew of it and used it medicinally centuries before us. It was first introduced to this country in the 16th century and seems to have had a mixed reception. Folklore said that once it was growing if you transplanted or uprooted parsley some disaster would befall you. In the Black Country parsley was always sown on a Good

Friday as it is difficult to germinate and it was said it went to the Devil and back several times before coming up!

In excess and as an oil it is extremely toxic and was once used as an **abortificant**. However, the amount we use in a garnish or a parsley sauce to pep up a bit of boring fish will do us good as it is rich in vitamins A and C, reduces inflammation and clears toxins.

Nettle rash was cured by rubbing with fresh parsley.

An old Leeds railwayman swore by parsley as a cure for **rheumatism**.

In Leicestershire they used a parsley **poultice** to cure a **stye**.

Water in which parsley had been boiled was drunk for **kidney complaints**.

Chewing parsley moistened with a little **vinegar** was said to get rid of **bad breath**.

An old beauty tip for clearing **spots** in a fortnight. Rub the spots with a dry cloth and then wash with rain water in which parsley has soaked overnight. This should be done 3 times a day.

PENNYROYAL. *Mentha pulegium* – a member of the mint family. A bitter, astringent herb used internally for **colds**, **whooping cough**, **indigestion** and for stimulating the uterus in menstrual complaints. See **menses**. An excess was taken as an **abortificant**.

An **infusion** of pennyroyal was a popular home remedy and in addition the leaves were the mystery ingredient in many North Country black puddings. In Warwickshire pennyroyal was picked in the fields and used to soothe colic in babies. It was also drunk to prevent deteriorating eyesight due to **diabetes**.

It was used for treating the whole family without men realising its many female uses – these things were not talked of openly. One elderly lady told me that she and her mother always had to smile when her father felt a cold coming on and asked for a brew of pennyroyal.

PENNYWORT. *Umbilicus rupestris*. Found growing on rocks, crevices and walls. Also called penny-pies by the gypsies who at one time mixed the leaves with animal fat and made a healing **ointment** for **wounds**.

PEONY. *Paeonia officinalis*. The root of the common peony was once a popular plant used medicinally in the Middle Ages. It has sedative properties and relaxes spasms. John Wesley in his *Primitive Physic* recommended the root for treating **epilepsy**.

PEPPERMINT. *Mentha x piperita*. Widely known and used for **indigestion** and for the relief of a **cold**. It was a popular drink prepared as a tea and its antispasmodic, expectorant and antiseptic properties were very useful for home medical remedies.

PERUVIAN BARK. Another name for the bark of the South American cinchona tree from which **quinine** was first extracted for the treatment of **malaria**.

PESTHOUSE. The 12th century forerunner of the isolation hospital, built outside the town, surrounded by a high wall, where people were taken with infectious diseases, most notably **leprosy**. As this disease declined it became a place where those suffering from the **plague** were taken. Pesthouses were there to protect those outside rather than treat the sick inside.

PESTILENT WORT. Once also known as plaguewort these were very old names for sweet coltsfoot, a closely allied species to the common **coltsfoot**. Found growing on the graves of those who had died from the **plague**, so desperate were people that it was taken as a sign to use the plant medicinally for treating the disease.

PHTHISIS. See **tuberculosis**.

PICK-ME-UP. An informal expression used by people when they were feeling a bit low and in need of some energy. A late 1800s **commonplace book** recorded rose petals soaked in whisky or wine. After 2 days, the undissolved bits were removed and it was ready to drink. This looks to me like a roundabout way of having a drop of alcohol and calling it medicine!

PILES. Or Haemorrhoids. To maintain regularity of the **bowels** and thus avoid the undue strain of **constipation** was known to be helpful with this condition. To that end a teaspoon of **senna** was recommended along with gall ointment night and morning. This ointment was made at home by mixing 2 ounces of lard, a pennyworth of **opium** and half an ounce of gall (a parasitic growth on a plant).

People were advised to replace the newspaper squares in the outside privy with proper bought lavatory paper The first lavatory paper, as we know it, did not appear until 1857, so the softer **dock leaf** must have been a preferred option. I was fascinated to learn that Henry VIII used sea shells for wiping the royal bottom, so for all his ill health in later years, piles were not one of his problems.

A common homemade **electuary** for piles was 1 ounce of **flowers of sulphur**, half an ounce of cream of tartar and some treacle mixed into a paste and taken 3 times a day.

John Wesley in *Primitive Physic* gave a list of substances to apply to the pile, none of which would appeal to us today.
'Apply warm treacle.'
'A Tobacco-leaf steep'd in water 24 hours.'
'A bruised Onion skin'd; or roasted in ashes.'
'Leeks fried in Butter.'
You might be forgiven for thinking you had slipped into a cookery book!

In my childhood you were warned never to sit on a cold surface as you would 'catch' piles, although sitting in flowing cold spring water was an old remedy for shrinking them – and much else besides. See also **pilewort**, **ulcer** and **wood betony**.

PILEWORT. *Ranunculus ficaria* or the lesser celandine. This plant is a good example of the **Doctrine of Signatures**, as the tubers on the root supposedly bear a resemblance to piles – a fact I cannot verify having never seen one. Known as pilewort by medieval medics it was widely used to treat this uncomfortable complaint. In fact the pilewort does have astringent properties so they were not that wide of the mark. The juice from the root was also used to cure **warts** and the young leaves with their vitamin C were eaten to prevent **scurvy**.

PIMPERNEL. *Anagallis arvensis*. Also known as scarlet pimpernel and poor man's weatherglass. A plant used for centuries in medicine for **vertigo** but now recognised as unsafe due to its powerful irritant and toxic properties.

PIMPLES. Taking a little **flowers of sulphur** powder before breakfast was recommended for minor blemishes. This had the effect of stimulating the **bowels**, sluggishness in which being seen as the root of most problems.

A 1930s home remedy book thought pimples were often caused by 'Excessive eating or drinking which the liver objects to.'

See also **spots**.

PISSE PROPHET. For centuries medical men and **quacks** relied on examining **urine** in order to give a diagnosis. In the 18th century a further diagnostic technique was refined whereby the doctor tasted the urine. This may seem repugnant to us now but it was a useful way of detecting **diabetes** as the urine tasted sweet. The urine in a glass bottle, called a jordan, was held up to the light and one can imagine the sucking of teeth and nodding of head as the poor victim was bamboozled by this show of learning and science.

PLACENTA. In isolated country areas some women ate the cooked placenta immediately after childbirth to prevent **post natal depression**. It was also used as a dressing on **ulcers** and rubbed

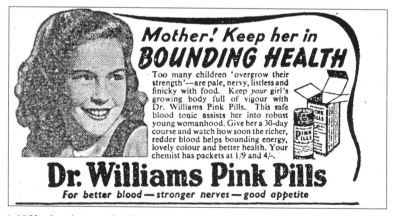

Mother! Keep her in
BOUNDING HEALTH

Too many children 'overgrow their strength'—are pale, nervy, listless and finicky with food. Keep *your* girl's growing body full of vigour with Dr. Williams Pink Pills. This safe blood tonic assists her into robust young womanhood. Give her a 30-day course and watch how soon the richer, redder blood helps bounding energy, lovely colour and better health. Your chemist has packets at 1/9 and 4/-.

Dr. Williams Pink Pills
For better blood — stronger nerves — good appetite

A 1952 advertisement for Pink Pills – a tonic containing iron. Many women still remember taking Pink Pills for Pale People in the 1940s and 1950s.

onto the mother's breast to prevent the nipples cracking while breast feeding. Whatever we might think of this now, undoubtedly there is a lot of goodness in a placenta.

In 19th century Cheshire a more sinister use was made of the placenta by men who thought they could capture a woman's heart by burying a placenta near her front door. Quite the reverse I should think!

PLAGUE. See **Black Death, bubonic plague, pestilent wort** and **Eyam**.

PLAGUE STONES. Sometimes known as Penny Stones or Vinegar Stones. An early form of disinfecting. I have found particular references to these stones in Cumbria, Kent, Lancashire, Yorkshire, Derbyshire, Shropshire, Cheshire and Northumberland.

The hollowed out stones, placed at the edge of a village suffering from the **plague**, contained water and **vinegar** and the villagers placed money in them to pay for supplies brought to them by outsiders. See also **Eyam**.

PLASTER. Or an older alternative spelling 'plaister'. A plaster was made at home by applying a substance, with some medicinal properties, to a piece of cloth and this was then put on to the painful part.

In the industrial towns of Lancashire a pitch plaster, a form of **tar**, was worn on the chest as a matter of course to keep clear of all chest infections. See also **mustard**.

PLEURISY. Inflammation of the pleura which separates the lungs from the chest, making breathing painful. Warmth was comforting and to that end **mustard** powder and water mixed and spread onto a wool flannel was placed onto the painful area.

In Cornwall during the First World War, Belgian refugees introduced the idea of a cat's skin placed on the chest for warmth when suffering from pleurisy. As a nation of animal lovers we may not have taken to this idea: we preferred a rabbit skin.

Far more pleasant for treating pleurisy was an **infusion** of **elderflowers** for drinking as tea.

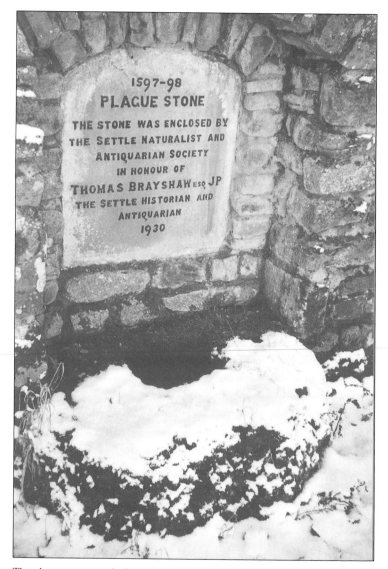

The plague stone on the boundary of Settle, North Yorkshire. The small trough once held vinegar and water in which villagers placed coins for goods received from outside the village. It was a primitive method of disinfecting and containing the infection. (Photograph Joy Calvert)

PNEUMONIA. An acute inflammation of the lungs caused by a bacterial or virus infection which before the advent of antibiotics was extremely serious, frequently leading to death. It was sometimes referred to as 'the old man's friend' as it was often responsible for a slow slipping away into death before the original illness killed you.

Standard home treatment got the patient into the kitchen with all the pans boiling to create steam to help with the breathing.

Either a hot **bread poultice** or a **kaolin poultice** was applied to the painful area of the chest. As an example of how little could be done before antibiotics I was told of an old doctor who was highly regarded by his patients. In cases of pneumonia he would visit every day and people thought his treatment was first rate. In fact all he did was move the poultice from one area of the chest to another! However you have to acknowledge that his visit would have brought great comfort to the distressed family.

From Wiltshire comes a more complicated **poultice** for pneumonia of 6 chopped **onions** added to some rye meal and enough **vinegar** to form a paste. This mixture was simmered for 10 minutes and put in large cotton bags and applied to the chest as hot as possible. After 10 minutes you replaced the bag with another one and you kept this up for a few hours until it was thought the patient was out of danger.

A drop of alcohol was a relaxant and one teaspoon 3 times a day from half a noggin of brandy with some **saffron** dissolved in it was said to be good for pneumonia.

PNEUMONIA JACKET. This was an article that 'old wives' insisted on when treating pneumonia. First the back and chest had a thick layer of **goose grease**, Vick or lard rubbed on. The jacket was a roll of cotton wool or flannel, cut into two pieces and held at the shoulders by two safety pins. Every morning a 1 inch strip was cut from the bottom of the jacket until it was all gone, by which time you were cured. Dire warnings were issued to those who had the cutting responsibility for if you removed it all at once the patient would go into a state of shock. Even in 1960 such was the power of these tales that a modern mother still heeded the advice

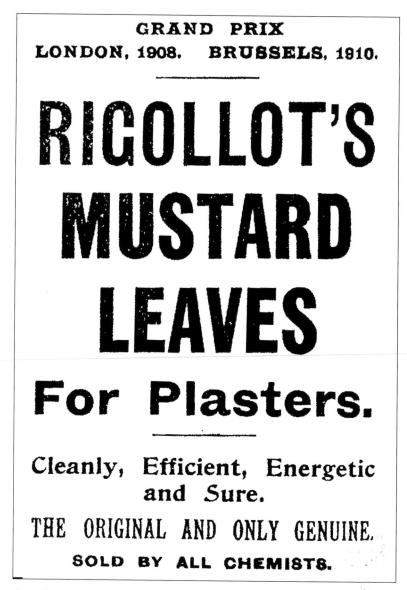

An early 1900s advertisment for mustard leaves to make your own mustard plaster which would have been heated and placed on the chest or painful part.

of the old lady next door and faithfully carried out the instructions on her young son to the letter.

POLIOMYELITIS. Otherwise known as Infantile Paralysis. This is an infectious disease of the spine and brain leading to paralysis or weakness in the limbs. The most serious cases were when the muscles used in breathing were affected and the patient was put into the 'iron lung' for artificial respiration.

For those born from the 1930s onwards, diseases such as **cholera** and **typhoid** are as much a part of history as the **plague**. The disease our parents most feared for us was polio and there were health warnings that at times of epidemics children should not go to crowded places like cinemas and swimming baths. Those with cautious mothers were never allowed to go to a swimming bath under any circumstances and a whole generation grew up not able to swim.

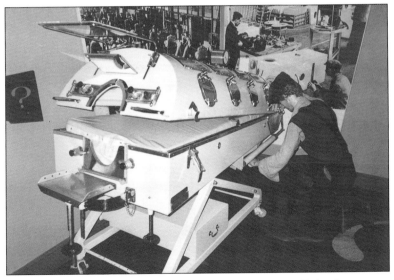

A Smith-Clarke ventilator, known as an 'Iron lung' for those suffering from poliomyelitis who needed artificial respiration. In the 1930s the great British manufacturer and philanthropist William Morris (1877–1963), later to become Lord Nuffield, gave over a car production line in the Cowley, Oxford plant of Morris Motors to making iron lung machines, which he gave free to hospitals. (By kind permission of the Thackray Museum, Leeds)

Polio is an old disease but epidemics were only recorded from the late 1800s onwards. Vaccination against polio started in the 1950s from a vaccine developed by Jonas Edward Salk. In 1956 there were 3,200 cases of polio; by the late 1960s the number was down to 24.

POPPY. *Papaver somniferum*. The opium poppy. Native annual herb of the Middle East and Asia but introduced and now naturalised throughout Europe where it is illegal to grow it without government permission. All parts are extremely poisonous. See also **opium**, **teething** and **toothache**.

PORRIDGE. See **oatmeal**.

POSSET. A drink of hot milk made to curdle by adding beer and flavoured with spices, once drunk as a remedy for a **cold**.

POST NATAL DEPRESSION. This was recognised but not treated in any way we would find acceptable now. *On the Diseases of Females* dated 1841 advised a variety of remedies from **blisters**, **purgatives** and a **mustard poultice** to the legs and thigh, 'Especially when great confusion in the head is present.' If none of these lifted the depression, 'The strait-waistcoat must be used without delay.'

In country areas, where they did without professional medical advice, the mother ate a mixture of ale, **oatmeal**, sugar and spices for several weeks after the birth to lift the spirits.

See also **placenta**.

POULTICE. A paste or soft mixture, generally hot, placed between 2 pieces of muslin or gauze and applied to the surface of the body. A poultice was used to soothe pain and where there was pus helped the formation of an abcess. A poultice softens the part of the body to which it is applied, dilates the blood vessels and increases the circulation.

A hot poultice is not suitable for swelling caused by a **sprain**, instead a cold poultice of **comfrey** should be used. Often a poultice was the only form of treatment available and everyone knew how to make one. They were in general use right up until the 1960s when modern medicine superseded this kind of treatment.

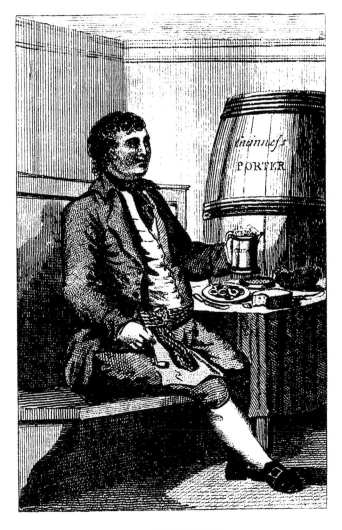

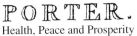

PORTER.
Health, Peace and Prosperity

From *The Gentleman's Magazine* of 1794 reflecting the 18th century view, which was probably correct, that Porter was safer and healthier to drink than water. The dark sweet ale brewed from black malt was originally known as Porter's ale because it was a favourite drink of porters.

The most common form of poultice was a **bread poultice**. Other popular ones were made from **soap** and sugar to draw out a splinter or 'spell'.

A poultice of **poppy** heads and **chamomile** flowers bought from a herbalist was used to draw **boils**.

For a collection of **boils**, known as a **carbuncle**, the more powerful **linseed** poultice was applied.

POWKE. Dialect word for **stye**.

PREGNANCY MYTHS. 'Old wives' came into their own when there was a pregnancy in the neighbourhood. If the mother put on weight all round her body it meant a boy, only at the front, a girl.

You could also predict the sex by holding a length of cotton over the mother's 'bump' and if it remained still the baby would be a girl and if it moved, a boy. One assumes this reflected the popular belief that as children boys were active and girls placid and still.

The pregnant mother should only look on beautiful things so that the child will also be beautiful!

Only the most virile men had daughters.

PRIMROSE. *Primula vulgaris*. All parts of the primrose were used for centuries in medicine. The plant contains saponins and aspirin

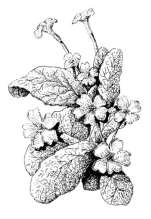

Primrose

like properties and it was used as an expectorant and for relaxing spasms. Primrose tea was used to treat **dysentery**.

PRUNES. Euphemistically known as 'little black coated workers' and held in high regard still as an **aperient**.

PUBLIC HANGING. If the felon was cut down from the gibbet still twitching the hands were thought to possess magical healing powers. There would be a surge of women all trying to press the dead man's hand against the parts needing healing. **Goitre, warts** and **wens** were singled out for this bizarre treatment.

The hand was cut off and embalmed with the fingers bent to hold a candle and in Yorkshire the 'hand of glory' was used by criminals to bring them luck as they went about their business. Not altogether successfully one imagines, as some believed holding the hand made them invisible!

After 1752 an Act of Parliament ordered the corpses to be delivered to a surgeon for public dissection. Not really as an act of public enlightenment and learning, more a deterrent. People believed that a spirit was condemned to limbo unless the body had a proper burial. Dissection was seen as a fate worse than death.

So adding to the ghastly scene round the gibbet was the unseemly scrum of those seeking a cure, the criminal's relatives fighting the medics for the body and the hangman, as part of the perks of the trade, trying to remove the corpse's clothes to sell. In parts of the West Country even the rope used for the hanging was cut up and sold as a talisman for people to wear in a bag round the neck, in the belief it would keep them well.

PUERPERAL FEVER. Also known as childbirth fever or childbed fever. The dangerous time was the second or third day after birth and it was the major cause of death to women after childbirth as at this time the woman was particularly susceptible to streptococcus infection. The complications were the same as for any infected wound, starting with fever and a raised temperature followed by inflammation, abscesses, peritonitis and at its worst septicaemia. Before sulphonamide drugs and penicillin death was inevitable.

The women were more often than not infected by those who

attended them during the birth, be it a doctor, midwife or neighbour. Hygiene was not understood and the midwife might well come direct from another birth without washing her hands, wearing the same blood-spattered clothes.

Little could be done until antiseptic procedures were adopted. In 1841 a doctor wrote that in the case of childbed fever he found helpful: '2 or 3 dozen **leeches** applied to the lower part of the belly. **Purgatives** – bowels must be strictly attended to.'

Even someone as comfortably placed and well organised as Mrs Beeton died aged 28, of puerperal fever following the birth of her fourth child in 1865.

PURGATIVE. A substance that causes a violent action of the **bowels** and stronger than an **aperient** or laxative. **Jalap** and scammony, a resin from the root of *Convolvulus scammonia*, a plant native to Turkey and Syria, were two of the most powerful purgatives. At one time they were called 'Drastics' and rightly so for you meant business if you took them. See also **aloes**.

PUSSY WILLOW. *Salix discolor.* An American willow tree with silvery catkins. In the latter part of the 19th century a **decoction** of the bark was drunk as an **aphrodisiac**.

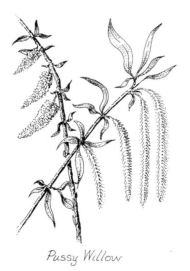

Pussy Willow

Q

Loss of Wealth is much; loss of Health is more.

QUACKS. In the 18th and 19th centuries uneducated people were at the mercy of travelling charlatans and con artists. In part John Wesley's *Primitive Physic* allowed ordinary people to have the knowledge to attempt some healing for themselves.

Quacks moved from town to town selling at fairs and markets, often with great showmanship. Dressing up as an American Indian or from the 'mysterious East' always added weight to the claims for their **nostrums**. Promoted with enough confidence any coloured liquid was bought by the gullible and desperate: in America they first coined the term 'snake oil' salesman. Some combined herbal mixtures with star signs and a reading of the constellations, others offered pieces of paper with a garbled extract from the Bible and amulets of dead bits of animals to hang round the neck, most contained **laudanum**.

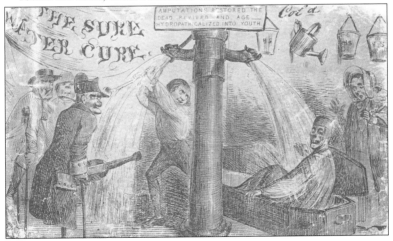

A Victorian cartoon from *Amusing Works* by Messrs Fores of Picadilly, showing the foolishness of those who believed in 'quack' medicines and the claims of some of the water cures. The sign on the pump reads, 'Amputations restored, the dead revived and age hydropathigalized into youth.' (By kind permission of Harrogate Museums and Art Gallery Service)

It is unfair to label all the suppliers of homemade ointments and potions as quacks for some supplied their local community and their remedies must have had a degree of success, otherwise people would not have gone back for more. Perhaps these concoctions worked because people wanted them to, or they would have got better anyway and the mixture did not actually do any harm.

For example, in Ambleside in Cumbria, a herb beer known as Black Drop was renowned as a good cure-all and a woman in Kendal, calling herself 'Mother Superior', provided toothache drops and powders for fractious babies. These preparations would undoubtedly have contained liberal doses of **laudanum**.

In the Black Country there were two well known local medicines, very highly regarded, called 'Draw it out' and 'Heal it up'.

A superstition found throughout England was that a woman who married but did not change the initial of her surname would have bad luck but would be able to heal others. Such women were sought out in country areas and asked for healing – no doubt money changed hands!

QUASSIA. A bitter compound extracted from the bark of a tree found in the West Indies, *Picraena excelsa*. It was named after the slave Graman Quassi who discovered its medicinal properties in the 18th century.

Quassia chips were in many medicine cupboards as they were a bitter tonic and used in convalescence to stimulate digestion and also as a **laxative**.

They were also used as a fly killer. A 1920s home remedy book advised that quassia chips with boiling water poured over them 'is a well known poison for flies'. This may also explain why some cases of head lice, popularly known as **nits,** were treated in the same way with quassia chips dissolved in hot water.

QUICK LIME. Calcium oxide. See **lime**.

QUICKSILVER. Another name for mercury. Apothecaries sold quills filled with quicksilver to help to fight illness – and if you were so troubled, it was useful against witches.

See also **vomiting**.

QUININE. A powerful antiseptic used in the treatment of **malaria** or **ague** as it destroys the malarial parasite in the blood. It was first extracted from the bark of the South American cinchona tree by the native Indians who knew centuries ago that it was effective in treating a fever. The tree was named after the Countess of Cinchon, the wife of the Spanish Viceroy of Peru, who brought the remedy to Europe in 1641 after being treated successfully with an **infusion** of the bark.

It was also called 'Jesuits' bark', after the Jesuits who learned of its healing uses from the natives and who offered the powdered bark as a treatment for ague in Europe. Anti-Catholic feeling and hysteria in England was so great at the time that the bark was shunned at first, but by the latter part of the 17th century it was being widely used.

Small amounts can act as a stimulating tonic and Edward Brown the Wensleydale farmer was recommending it back in 1895 for **nervous disorders**. Tonic water contains quinine and must have been so called because of its beneficial qualities. In view of the medicinal properties of **gin** and the quinine in tonic, a small gin and tonic probably ought to be available on prescription!

QUINSY. A complication leading on from **tonsillitis** where an **abscess** forms under the mucous membrane surrounding the tonsils, making it painful to swallow, speak and open the mouth.

John Wesley in *Primitive Physic* accurately described quinsy as 'A fever attended with difficulty of swallowing and often breathing', but his advice, so often helpful, would in this case only make the patient look rather silly, 'Apply a large White-bread toast, half an inch thick, dipt in Brandy to the crown of the head 'till it dries.'

Slightly less odd and of some comfort and a remedy used many times throughout the country was heated **salt** put in a stocking and wrapped round the neck.

Every Housewife's Guide Book, a publication much valued for its advice during the Second World War, recommended a rubbing **liniment** for quinsy. 1 ounce each of **turpentine**, liquid ammonia and **olive oil** mixed together and applied with a flannel to the throat.

The leaves from red **sage** were made into an **infusion** and used as a gargle for quinsy.

The juice or the jelly from **blackcurrant**, once known as the quinsy berry, or a **decoction** from the leaves or bark was astringent and soothing.

If you could manage it, sipping Worcester sauce was said to be very effective for the relief of quinsy.

R

Early to bed and early to rise, makes a man healthy, wealthy and wise.

RABBIT SKIN. Placed on the chest in cases of **pleurisy** for warmth, a rabbit skin provided a more comfortable option than **brown paper**. At one time there was a plentiful supply of rabbits for the poor to trap and eat. All country people could skin a rabbit, and when I was a child, as in many other homes, our larder was seldom without a hanging dead rabbit.

A leaflet issued by the National Federation of Women's Institutes dated 1951 instructed its members on how to cure the skin of a rabbit, lamb, mole or goat using powdered alum and salt. I doubt the Women's Institute would feel the need for such a leaflet now.

RABIES. See **mad dog bite** and **rose hips**.

RASPBERRY. *Rubus idaeus*. This plant has been used in herbal medicines for centuries as its astringent properties are helpful in stomach upsets and **diarrhoea**.

Taken in small doses in the last few weeks of pregnancy – but never at the beginning – raspberry leaf tea is still used to aid childbirth contractions as it tones the uterus.

Raspberrry vinegar was very good for **colds** and **sore throats**.

Raspberry Vinegar

Put 4 lbs 8 ounces of raspberries in a bowl and pour over 3 pints of white vinegar, cover with a cloth and leave for 48 hours. Strain and boil the juice with 1 lb of sugar for each pint of juice. Bring to the boil and then simmer gently. Keep skimming the surface until perfectly clear. Cool and bottle.

RED OIL. *The Housewife's Friend and Family Help* in the early 1900s referred to: 'This valuable article. . . for bruised or sore feet, caused by rubbing of the boot or shoe, nothing can be better than this.' The oil was made from the flowers and stems of

St John's Wort soaked in a bottle of **olive oil** left on a window sill in the sun for about 6 weeks and then strained. The oil got its name from the red pigment of the crushed flowers.

RHEUMATISM. Any ache or stiffness was called 'rheumatics' in the past. The length of this entry shows the problem it must have been, with remedies ranging from the commonsense to the bizarre – but if it worked for you, who cared.

Many of the **commonplace books** I read while researching this book had any number of references to rheumatism. Those who suffered were desperate for some pain relief and remedies and ideas were passed round. Keeping warm and out of draughts, sleeping only in well aired beds and wearing plenty of warm underwear with a layer of **flannel** were all part of the fight against rheumatism. See also **laudanum**.

For those who could afford it a trip to a delightful **spa** town for a Turkish Bath or one of the many rich and varied water treatments.

An optimistic cure found in an old **commonplace book** from the late 1800s, belonging to a lady who was born in Louth, Lincolnshire and moved to Hebden Bridge, Yorkshire in 1890 to be 'in service'. 'We have given this prescription to scores of friends and not had one failure. You need 3 grapefruit, 3 oranges, 3 lemons. 2 ounces each of **Epsom salts** and cream of tartar. Squeeze the juice from all the fruits and set aside. Put all skins, pulp and seeds through a mincer and pour 2 pints of boiling water over this. Add the fruit juice and let it stand overnight. Next day extract all the juice by squeezing through a fine sieve or cloth. Dissolve the cream of tartar and Epsom salts in 1 pint of boiling water and add to the juice. Bottle and keep in a cool place. Take 1 wineglass before breakfast each day – only one dose a day. Keep this up for 27 weeks, by which time the system will have thrown off all stiffness of the joints.'

Another old remedy dating from the same time recommended drinking plenty of water in which either **parsley** or celery had been boiled, or alternatively suggested eating the outer layer of the celery, the bit that is normally thrown away.

A mild **aperient** using **lemons** was always thought of as helpful.

Homemade **embrocation** and **liniment** in the **rubbing bottle** was eagerly applied. Other external treatments included wrapping a **vinegar** bandage or a wash leather round a painful knee or the more pleasant warm treacle smeared onto **brown paper**.

Or you could apply a **poultice** of boiled bay leaves or **horseradish**.

Another suggestion was to hold the afflicted joint over the steam when cooking **cabbage**. Not suitable for the hips for obvious reasons.

Common soda was dissolved in hot water and vigorously rubbed onto the painful part.

You were often advised to wear sheepswool next to the skin.

Other remedies believed to work but not perhaps with any science behind them:

Sleep with a cork under the pillow at night.

Wear a strand of worsted or knitting wool round the wrist.

Always carry any of the following in your pocket: a potato, a **nutmeg**, a piece of ashwood, a lump of **brimstone**.

To this day some people swear by wearing a copper bangle.

Carry a powerful magnet or attach one to the foot of the bed.

In Cumbria they believed wearing the skin of an eel wrapped round an arm or a leg would help. An added bonus was that the eel skin offered protection from getting rheumatism in the first place. If not available a more difficult option was carrying a live toad somewhere on the person. If it could be managed a bee sting on the rheumatic part was said to give some relief.

Items I came across supposed to be good for relieving rheumatism were: white **bread**, **coltsfoot**, **dandelion** leaves, **garlic**, **honey**, **rhubarb**, **sneezewort**, **sweet cicely**, **tar water**, **turpentine** and **yarrow** tea. Take your pick there must be something there for you!

RHEUM. An old term for a watery discharge from the eyes or nose.

RHUBARB. *Rheum*. Rhubarb was grown at one time in most English gardens and eaten extensively in puddings and jam. The stalks have many useful medicinal properties as a stimulant to digestion and as a **purgative**.

See also **Turkey rhubarb** and **Indian brandee**.

Many people recall urine from the chamber pot put onto the garden soil to make the rhubarb stalks particularly succulent. Not everyone viewed this as a good thing and one old lady told me that she always refused the neighbour's offer: 'Do have some rhubarb – it's good and juicy now.'

This reminds me of the old story of the elderly gentleman out in the road following a horse and cart and shovelling up the horse manure. A little boy watching him asked, 'What do you need that for?' and the old man answered, 'I put it on my rhubarb.' The little boy replied, 'We put custard on ours.'

RICKETS. Right up until the late 1950s many children from poor families in industrial towns were afflicted by this disease. The restricted diet and lack of both milk and sunshine caused a deficiency in vitamin D and young growing bones became soft and malformed.

In the past, vitamins were not understood any more than the action of ultra-violet light in converting the skin fats to vitamin D. However, it was clear that even 18th century doctors knew it was linked to a poor diet. Maximilian Hazlemore in 1794 wrote, 'Good claret mixed with equal quantity of water. Those who cannot afford claret, may give the child now and then a wineglass of mild ale or good porter. The diet ought to be dry and nourishing, as good bread, roasted flesh etc.'

He also firmly believed that 'Children begotten by men in the decline of life who are subject to the gout, the gravel or other chronic diseases are liable to the ricketts [sic].'

John Wesley in *Primitive Physic* could only suggest **cold baths** as a cure and it is interesting to see that 150 years later no cure was offered in the many home remedy books, but there was the advice: 'Ablutions is a very important preventative.' In the 1950s children at risk of rickets were sent for a weekly dose of 'sun ray' treatment.

It was a very old superstition that cutting the inside of the child's ear would cure rickets.

Somerset folklore believed rubbing the child's body with snails cured rickets.

RINGWORM. A highly contagious fungus infection that was once a common sight, especially on the head but it can affect other parts of the body. It spread like wildfire in schools and institutions. Now it is treated with antifungal cream or antibiotics but once the juice of the **houseleek** or a **decoction** of **soapwort** was thought effective.

Other kitchen cupboard remedies used a layer of treacle on the patches of ringworm, a mixture of ink and **onion**, which would have really drawn attention to the problem or an ointment made from **pennyroyal** and lard.

In Shropshire the grease, called bletch, from the church bells was thought a useful treatment.

In highly superstitious remote country areas people believed 'charmers' could clear ringworm by muttering incantations, just as in curing **warts**.

By the 1900s a home remedy book recommended matches, presumably because of the **sulphur** content. 'A very simple cure is to dip the ends of a number of matches in water, and apply the ends of the matches daily to the spot.'

See also **athlete's foot**.

ROBIN-RUN-IN-HEDGE. See **Ground Ivy**.

ROSE HIPS. Produced on the wild dog rose, *Rosa canina*. As a child in Cumbria I was out with a tin bowl and a walking stick in early autumn, eagerly picking the rose hips from the farmers' hedges. The hips were for commercial use and the collection point was the village post office. There the postmistress weighed them and you were paid, sadly I cannot remember how much, and if you picked a large amount there was an added incentive of a badge! Rose hips are rich in vitamins B and C and rose hip tea is a

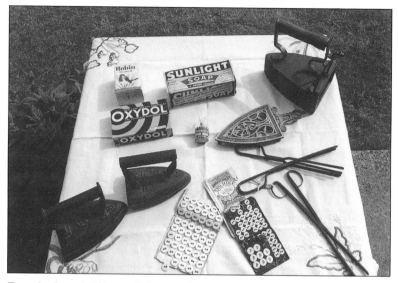

Everyday household items. Robin starch was not only responsible for a stiff, starched collar but was also used dry as a cure for chapped hands and on a baby's bottom for nappy rash. The Reckitt's Blue bag whitened clothes and was dabbed on stings, leaving a tell-tale blue mark. Sunlight soap washed both clothes and the skin. The heated flat irons helped with backache. (Photograph Ann Holubecki)

tonic as well as having diuretic properties. It was drunk in cases of exhaustion and convalescence and to guard against **colds**. Rose hip syrup was given to babies and for a **cough**.

The dog rose was so called because of the mistaken belief that the roots would cure **rabies**.

ROSEMARY. *Rosmarinus officinalis*. An aromatic restorative herb rich in oils and used for centuries in medicine. The root was part of a long list of herbs used to make **plague** water. Rosemary has always been associated with remembrance as in: 'There's rosemary, that's for remembrance,' Shakespeare's *Hamlet*. Recently there have been claims that it will help prevent loss of memory as we grow old.

The young fresh leaves and flowers can be dried and used for **decoctions**, **infusions** and **tinctures**. Herbalists used it for many complaints including **tuberculosis** as it relaxes, relieves pain, stimulates the **liver** and **gall bladder** and is good for the digestion.

Everyone knows about rosemary, even if only for flavouring the roast lamb. Why then did I fail to find it mentioned in any home remedies? It does not seem to have been part of everyday family medicine, John Wesley in *Primitive Physic* mentioned it for **earache**. Originally it came from the Mediterranean and thrives in dry, warm, sheltered areas, not the climate to describe England; perhaps many people just could not grow it in the past.

ROYAL BLOOD MIXTURE. Quoted in a 1920s home remedy book as a famous **specific**. 'A miraculous medicine for all Blood Diseases; used in the Royal Navy for **scrofula**, **syphilis** and various Glandular Diseases, and effects cures even under the disadvantages of a salt meat diet on board ship.' The 'miraculous' ingredients were a small amount of potassium iodide, which caused absorption of unhealthy syphilitic tissues, and large amounts of **sarsaparilla**.

RUBBING BOTTLE An informal name given to the bottle in every home containing a 'rub' for relieving **rheumatism**. See also **liniment** and **embrocation**. The contents acted as a counter-irritant replacing a nasty pain with a nice warm one.

A very easy 'rub' to take the pain away temporarily was 2 ounces of chillies soaked in 5 fluid ounces of methylated spirits.

RUE. *Ruta graveolens*. Also known as the herb of grace. All parts of this plant are poisonous, although this did not stop people in the past drinking rue tea for stomach ache and giving cold rue tea first thing in the morning to stimulate a lazy child! Like **rosemary** the root was used in **plague** water and as a cure for **earache**.

Rue is highly dangerous for pregnant women as it stimulates the uterus and knowing this women took too much and used it as an **abortificant**. The plant was used in the past to increase lactation in nursing mothers and . . . cows.

It was made into posies and placed in the courtrooms to prevent the judges from catching gaol fever. See also **typhus**.

RUPTURE. Another name for hernia. For a rupture in a child John Wesley in *Primitive Physic* advised applying hot cow dung on leather to a 'windy rupture'. However, for an adult a mixture of

agrimony, Solomon's Seal and strawberry roots in white wine would cure in 2 weeks. He did offer more practical advice, 'A good Truss meantime is of great use.'

Superstitious country people in the 18th and 19th centuries claimed an unlikely cure for a hernia by passing a child from east to west through a split ash sapling. In some places a particular tree was kept permanently split with a wedge.

RUN DOWN. Written in a 1890s **commonplace book**, 'For Run down feeling' – and how we can sympathise, for 100 years on we still get that feeling from time to time. Here the writer recorded a simple recipe of twopence worth of gentian root, the root of the European yellow gentian and a bitter tonic herb, which she must have bought from a herbalist, and some orange and lemon peel. This was boiled all together with a pint of water and a wineglassful was recommended 3 times a day.

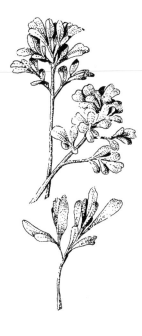

Rue

S

SAFFRON. *Crocus sativus.* The flower pistils have been used for centuries in medicine and for colouring. The medical properties of the plant stimulate the circulation and increase the perspiration. See also **jaundice** and **pneumonia**.

For a time saffron was grown at Saffron Walden in Essex where it was used as dye in the cloth and wool trade.

SAGE. *Salvia officinalis,* salvia from the Latin 'salvere' meaning 'to be in good health'. Sage has been used for centuries as a medicinal aid. It was traditionally associated with long life and was also planted on graves as it was thought to lessen grief.

Sage has antiseptic and anti inflammatory properties, relaxes spasms, increases **liver** function and aids digestion but like all things, too much for too long is bad for you.

Sage tea was said to be good for **dizziness**, the **palsy**, **sunburn**, restoring a failing memory in the old, and night sweats, especially in the **menopause**.

John Wesley in *Primitive Physic* advised, 'Boil white and red Sage, a handful of each in a quart of white wine. Strain and bottle it. Take a small glass morning and evening. This helps all nervous disorders.'

Washing hair in an **infusion** of sage was said to stop it falling out.

Sage leaves were also good to rub onto a bruise or you could clean your teeth with them.

We now associate sage with cooking as in sage and onion stuffing, flavouring sausages and the famous Sage Derby cheese.

ST ANTHONY'S FIRE. See **erysipelas**.

ST JOHN'S WORT. *Hypericum perforatum.* Visit any pharmacy or health food shop now and there will be racks of products containing St John's Wort; it is very much the 'wonder' herb of today. However, its healing properties have been known since medieval times. The red dots on the leaves were thought to look like wounds and the plant was used for healing in the Crusades by the Knights of St John of Jerusalem.

In folk medicine the plant was hung over doors to ward off evil spirits. It was also used in the treatment of depression and its sedative properties were useful in cases of disturbed sleep. It is now hailed as giving a boost to menopausal women.

ST VITUS'S DANCE. Also known as Sydenham's Chorea and related to rheumatic fever. The symptoms of involuntary twitching, jerking movements and loss of co-ordination led to the name 'dance'. In the Middle Ages people in certain parts of Germany were prone to mass hysteria, which took the form of manic dancing (I would imagine an all night 'rave' might be similar). They would pray at the chapels of St Vitus, a third century child martyr, who they believed would cure them. See also **epilepsy**.

Aspirin, steroids and rest would be prescribed now but for centuries **mistletoe** tea was the cure – and it might have been quite helpful.

SALIVA. Otherwise known as spit or spittle has powerful digestive enzymes and the first spit of the day was thought to be the strongest and was known as **fastin' spittle**. It was said to be very effective on a **stye**.

A mother will still 'kiss it better' when a child is hurt and unknowingly she is taking part in an age old belief, for which there is some substance. Human saliva contains a natural healing chemical lysozyme, which is why when you crush a **dock leaf** it should always have spit added for soothing a **sting**.

A dog's saliva was almost as good and many people still allow their dogs to lick a septic **cut**.

When doing housework or cleaning, the term 'spit and polish' was taken literally; cleaning with a good dollop of spit. There is scientific proof that human spit is a powerful cleaner, breaking down any fatty deposits on a dirty surface, although I think most

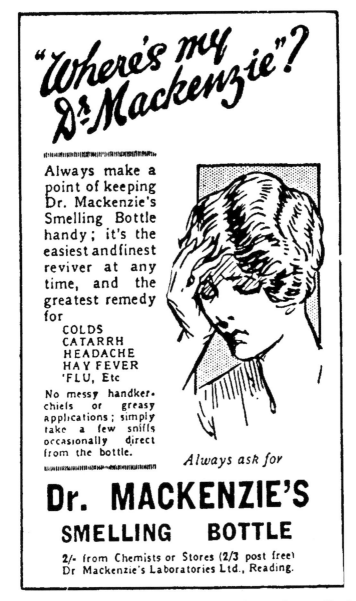

Does anyone carry smelling salts now? A 1931 advertisement for a smelling bottle which would have contained sal volatile.

of us would still prefer a can of spray polish.

SALT. Salt has been mined in Cheshire since 1670 and was a considerably healthier occupation than mining lead, coal, tin or copper.

From the Black Country Society's *Bostin' Fittle* by Pat Purcell, I found an interesting old use of salt for muscular aches. Pieces of rock salt were fried and placed inside a bag of Welsh flannel and then placed on a sore muscle or painful joint. You had another ready heating in the oven for when the bag cooled.

Common salt mixed with water required real courage to take but it was a very effective gargle for a **sore throat**. A dab of salt placed directly onto a mouth ulcer would result in exquisite agony for a few seconds but a marked shrinking of the ulcer. Salt mixed with soot was an effective, if abrasive toothpaste.

According to *Gray's Pharmacopoeia* of 1831 salt was used in medicine, 'In **clysters** as a purge', dissolved in water and drunk as a stimulant and in a lotion for a **wen** or bruising.'

See also **mad dog bite**, **sea bathing** and **sea water**.

SALTPETRE. Also known as **nitre**. In powder form it was a constituent of gunpowder and a preservative. An irritant to the stomach, it is unwise to take it internally but in the past it was part of an unusual treatment for **boils**. A remedy from the early 1900s, recommended by a doctor to a farmer, was to empty a shotgun cartridge and discard the lead shot and wadding but keep the black gunpowder separately. Each evening you took a glass of warm water and placed as much gunpowder as would lay on a sixpence and mixed this with the water. Drink this mixture on rising the next morning, you were told, and you would be cured in a few days.

SALVE. See **ointment**.

SAL VOLATILE. Aromatic spirit of ammonia and a powerful stimulant. See **hartshorn**.

SAMPHIRE. *Crithmum maritimum*. Also known as sea fennel and a plant very high in vitamin C. Once it grew abundantly along the

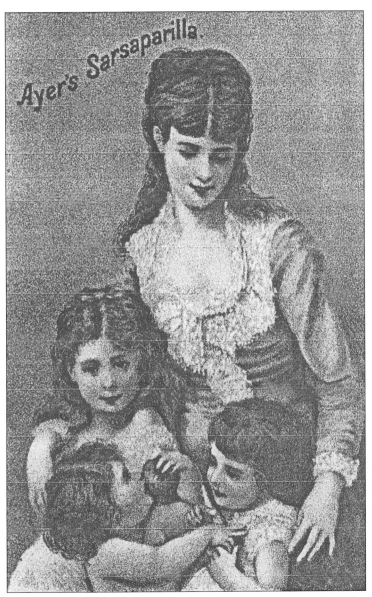

Ayer's Sarsaparilla included some iron and was a very popular non-alcoholic and non-addictive patent medicine that probably did some good. (By kind permission of the Thackray Museum, Leeds)

Sussex coast and was collected commercially and sold by apothecaries as a cure for **scurvy**.

SARSAPARILLA. A non-alcoholic drink prepared from the long, twisted sassafrass root of various Central American species of Smilax. It was generally combined with some iron and was a popular ingredient in patent medicines for 'purifying the blood.' For menopausal women in the 1900s it was the HRT treatment of its day and Ayer's Sarsaparilla was universally recommended for all problems associated with the **change of life**. It was the main ingredient in **Royal blood mixture**. See also **whites**.

SCABIES. Also known as the **itch**. A highly contagious condition that spread quickly in overcrowded and dirty conditions. It was a great problem in the British Army. Sleeping in a bed previously occupied by someone infected was a sure way of catching it. Scabies is caused by the mite *Sarcoptes scabiei* which burrows into the skin, leaving very itchy pimples, which then become infected when scratched. Dusting yourself with **sulphur** was a part cure.

SCALDS. A very common occurrence in families when all cooking and heating of water was done on the kitchen range. From a 1900s home remedy book: 'Place the part in **lime** water.' See also **burns**.

SCARBOROUGH. This bracing town on the east coast of Yorkshire styled itself the 'Queen of the Watering Places.' In 1620 Mrs Elizabeth Farrow discovered a spring near the south shore and declared the taste horrible enough to be medicinal. As well as drinking this water, Scarborough offered bathing in an invigorating North Sea environment and was in at the start of the **sea bathing** craze.

There was much rivalry between **Harrogate** and Scarborough as to which was the healthiest. Dr Charles Rooke of Scarborough became famous in the late 1800s for his medical pamphlets and patent remedies. Dr Rooke's Oriental Pills guaranteed to cleanse you of 'All unhealthy accumulations'.

SCARIFICATION. A once very popular method of **blood-letting** by making several small, shallow cuts in the skin to draw blood.

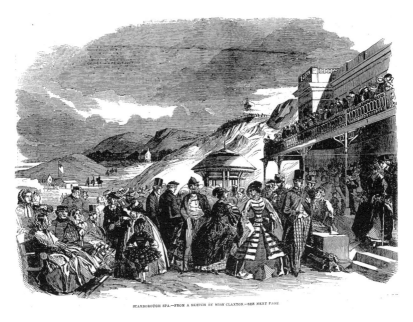

SCARBOROUGH SPA.—FROM A SKETCH BY MISS CLAXTON.—SEE NEXT PAGE.

Elegant society in Scarborough from *The Illustrated London News* of 1858. 'Its effects in debility arising from diseases of the stomach and digestive organs and on the kidneys are well known, and, in combination with pure bracing air and delightful seabathing, has made Scarborough the resort not only of all health and pleasure seekers in Yorkshire, but from all parts of the kingdom.'

SCARLET FEVER. An infectious disease which quickly spread out of control: even the clothes and belongings of those affected could be infectious. Malnourished children in poor and overcrowded homes were especially susceptible, as were women who had just given birth. It is a streptococcal infection so before the introduction of antibiotics all that could be done was to try and reduce the fever and soothe the sore throat and rash. Every large town had an isolation hospital to which patients would be taken.

People were rightly frightened of the disease and Mac Webster, a retired fireman provided me with this picture of life in Sheffield in the 1930s and 40s. 'The blue ambulance was the fever ambulance. People suffering from scarlet fever and **diphtheria** were moved to Lodge Moor outside Sheffield. People would keep away from the street where the sick person lived for a week. When you visited you stood on a verandah and waved at the patient through the window. It was very, very cold up there. People wore **iodine** lockets in Sheffield as they were supposed to stop you catching scarlet fever and diphtheria and they smelt terrible.'

If you had been in contact with someone with scarlet fever you went straight home and gargled with **salt** water.

SCIATICA. Intense pain down the sciatic nerve spreading from the buttocks down the thigh to the calf often caused by a prolapsed intervertebral disc. In the early 1900s **camphor** was dissolved in a pint of boiling water and a wineglassful drunk 3 times a day. Understanding what we do now of camphor this was not a good idea and was unlikely to have done any good.

Far nicer must have been the country cure of **elderberry** juice mixed with port wine. It is hard, however, to imagine how the remedy from rural Wiltshire, of two nutmegs in your pocket, might have worked.

John Wesley in *Primitive Physic* described the pain accurately but spoilt his diagnosis by claiming, 'The Sciatica is certainly cured by a **purge** taken in a few hours after it begins.' If this did not work his other vigorous approach was, 'Use cold bathing, and sweat, together with the flesh-brush twice a day.'

Various hot **poultices** were said to do the trick, especially one made of **nettles**. At least while you were applying the poultice you were resting and this was likely to have done you as much good as anything.

SCODER. Cumbrian dialect word for a friction 'sare' (sore) caused by the rubbing of heavy boots or clogs against the skin. The cure was to rub the inside of your socks with a mix of starch and boracic acid powder which would dry the sore and acted as an antiseptic.

SCROFULA. See **King's evil**, **Margate** and **Royal blood mixture**.

SCURVY. A disease caused by a lack of vitamin C over several months leading to **anaemia**, gum problems where the teeth drop out and bleeding beneath the skin. The appalling bad breath that accompanies all this seems a minor inconvenience.

John Wesley in *Primitive Physic* seemed to understand what was lacking in those suffering from scurvy. He advocated a diet of **turnips, horseradish, nettle** juice, **watercress, dock** roots, Sevil [sic] oranges and a pint of **lime** juice twice a day.

To keep scurvy at bay many preferred to eat the leaves of the common scurvy grass, *Cochlearia officinalis*, which is found by the sea or the vitamin rich **samphire**. See also **pilewort**.

Sailors were the obvious candidates for this illness but so too were soldiers away on campaigns and those in prison and the workhouse.

Captain James Cook (1728–79) is credited with understanding that a diet of fresh fruit and vegetables kept his sailors free of scurvy. In 1795 scurvy was beaten on board ship by the British Navy introducing a daily ration of lemon or **lime** juice giving rise to the name 'limeys'. The long passage by British immigrants to Australia led to the Aussie use of the word, not altogether kindly meant, to describe those seeking a new life.

SEA BATHING. In spite of the cold, sea bathing became very popular from the 1730s onwards, as a great tonic among the wealthier classes. **Brighton, Margate, Southend** and the chillier **Scarborough** were all fashionable sea bathing resorts. One hired a bathing hut which was wheeled into the sea, together with a male 'dipper' who lifted you into the water. In spite of women being amply covered there was much excited lewd comment among male loafers on the sea shore.

According to *Elements of Materia Medica and Therapeutics*, a paper written in 1832 by A. T. Thompson, sea bathing was a great aid to digestion and to the heart. On leaving the water even greater 'tone' could be achieved if you allowed yourself to dry naturally, leaving the salt particles on the skin.

Thompson also recommended sea bathing as a cure for **rheumatism** and catarrh, giving as an example Captain William Bligh (1754-1817) of HMS *Bounty*. Captain Bligh was a tough disciplinarian and the Mutiny was a complex affair but one gets a

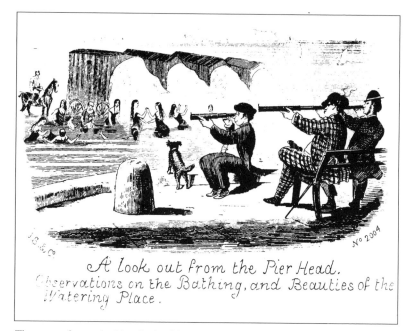

A look out from the Pier Head.
Observations on the Bathing, and Beauties of the
Watering Place.

The vogue for sea bathing for health reasons probably gave more pleasure to the
gentlemen on the shore than it did to those ladies emerging from the bathing
machines for an invigorating cold dip. From a wood engraving inscribed 'J.S.&
Co'. (The Wellcome Library, London)

glimpse of the man here. 'It has always been a remark of seamen,
that in dry weather neither rheumatism nor catarrhs are caught at
sea, however frequently the body may be wet with the spray or the
waves of the sea. Captain Bligh, who traversed an immense tract
of ocean, with 17 of his crew, in an open boat, preserved his
companions and himself from these diseases, although they were
exposed to frequent rains. He effected this by immersing the shirts
and jackets of the seamen in the sea water, and ordering them to
be worn in their moist state.'

He must have been a hard man to like.

SEA SICKNESS. Brown paper tucked under a foundation garment
was said to cure sea sickness and this method was still being used
up to the 1950s.

Others to this day still swear by **ginger** or a little drop of brandy.

An early 1900s home remedy book thought a substantial meal before going on board would help and once at sea a teaspoonful of cocoa in a little water every 2 hours.

The Northampton Living Memory Group reported that an easy, if unusual cure was to break an egg and remove the inner membrane, before setting off on your journey. The membrane was then rolled into a little ball and kept in the pocket. When you felt sea sick you swallowed the ball and on reaching the stomach, it unravelled and formed a protective lining.

SEA WATER. In 1754 Dr Richard Russell arrived in the little village of Brighthelmstone in Sussex, later to be known as Brighton. He soon achieved fame and a 'following' for his claims to cure most illnesses with either **sea bathing** or drinking sea water. His dissertation on *The use of Seawater in the diseases of the glands*, published in 1752 had been a great success.

So popular were his ideas that Brighton sea water was bottled and sold for drinking in London. The noxious brew of sea water boiled with milk and some cream of tartar, strained and cooled must have caused untold misery to those trying for a cure.

See also **eczema**, **Margate** and **shingles**.

SENNA. Responsible for so much misery as it was probably the number one favourite **aperient**. From the tropical species Cassia the leaves in tea form and the dried fruits or pods all produced the same effect.

Mrs Keenlyside's Spring Medicine

Into a large jug place 12 senna pods, 2 teaspoons of **Epsom salts**, the juice of a **lemon**, 1 flat teaspoon of cream of tartar, sugar to taste. **Infuse** in 3 pints of boiling water which has slightly cooled.

In one Yorkshire family a small glass of this was taken just before going to school!

SHIN. For a broken shin John Wesley advised in *Primitive Physic*: 'Bind a dry Oak-leaf upon it.'

SHINGLES. Painful blisters which form a ring round the body. Folk medicine believed that if the ring joined up you were about to die. There were two options for a cure – drinking **sea water** or an **infusion** of **blackberry** leaves – and I know which one I would have chosen.

SIMPLE. An old term for a herb used for healing purposes. The process of making up the cure was called 'simpling'.

SLEEPLESSNESS. A worker in the past would not have understood our current obsession with sleep for if you had put in 8 hours or more heavy manual work, you had little difficulty sleeping. Judging from newspaper articles and books on the subject, the search for a good night's sleep is an enduring one. If you have difficulty sleeping it becomes an obsession and we all know those who, at breakfast, feel it necessary to give a detailed account of every sleepless hour. Even the young have trouble sleeping now, in the past it would have been only the old. The older we become the less sleep we need at night but the urge for the so seductive afternoon nap becomes greater.

For those troubled by sleeplessness some advice from the past may be useful.

John Wesley in *Primitive Physic* called the inability to sleep 'Vigilia' and his advice was to have a cold bath or to apply water lily leaves to the head.

A century later 'The Lady's World' of 1898 recommended: 'A hot **mustard** footbath before going to bed. Heavy meals should be avoided, as should **tea**, **coffee** and alcoholic stimulants except for a couple of tablespoons of whisky taken with half a tumblerful of hot water before going to bed. In slight cases of insomnia most people will derive great benefit by taking a glass of ale or stout every night about half an hour before going to bed.'

The afternoon zizz is not all bad as a 1930s home remedy book believed that: '5 minutes' sleep is equal to 1 pound of beefsteak.'

Further comments on the subject of sleep from the same book claimed 1 hour's sleep before midnight was worth 3 after midnight and that early risers were long livers.

Some people thought eating a few grapes or taking a teaspoon of milk of magnesia in water just before going to bed helped you to sleep.

Other advice from the past ranged from attending to one's **bowels**, taking a 'sharp' walk before bedtime and sleeping with the windows open. See also **bread**, **hops** and **valerian**.

SLIPPERY ELM. The sterilised and washed outer bark of the red elm tree, *Ulmus rubra*, was used as an **abortificant**. It was inserted into the vagina and kept there for about 45 minutes. It was one of the methods used by urban back street abortionists and a safer method than the horrendous knitting needle. It is now subject to legal restriction in many countries. See also **menses**.

A less heroic side of how the West was won in America revealed the Native North Americans' use of slippery elm as an abortificant when there was the possibility of the baby being a half breed.

However, in powdered form slippery elm also has healing and laxative properties and was regarded as good for invalids when mixed with sugar and milk. Externally it was used in a **poultice** for treating a deep cut.

SMALLPOX. Once called the 'speckled monster' and a contagious and dreaded worldwide scourge for centuries. The fever and pus-filled blisters were accompanied by swelling, inflammation and an awful smell, and if you recovered, you were left with scars and possibly blindness. The World Health Organisation announced that smallpox had been eradicated only in the late 1970s.

In 17th century Restoration England the fashion for wearing patches on the face arose from the need to hide the smallpox scars. We are told that 1 in 5 deaths were caused by smallpox in the 18th century and the death rate was just as high in Victorian England.

In China and the East it had been the practice for centuries to take a small amount of pus from someone with a mild case of smallpox and use this to infect a healthy person, thereby giving them a mild dose and rendering them immune from further contagion. Lady Mary Wortley Montagu (1689–1762), the wife of the British Ambassador to Turkey, who herself was badly scarred by smallpox, brought back the idea to England in 1717, although it was not greeted with any enthusiasm until royalty gave it the seal of approval and had it done. Many opposed it on religious grounds seeing the illness as a punishment sent from God.

The only women having perfect complexions were milkmaids who had caught the milder cowpox and thereby had immunity from smallpox.

> 'Where are you going my pretty maid?
> I'm going a milking Sir, she said,
> What is your fortune my pretty maid?
> My face is my fortune Sir, she said.'

Inoculation by nicking the skin and passing a thread with smallpox pus on it was all a bit hit and miss and you were either lucky and had a slight dose or you developed full scale smallpox. The safer and more reliable cowpox vaccination was developed by Edward Jenner, a surgeon from Berkeley, Gloucestershire in 1796.

John Wesley in *Primitive Physic* thought drinking 'largely of Toast and Water' was helpful and further recommended a pint of cold water. 'This instantly stops the convulsions, and drives out the pock.'

The usual treatments were given as for a **fever** but in the case of smallpox applying cool, previously boiled **turnips** to the feet was recommended for bringing down the temperature.

An ointment made from charcoal and lard was said to prevent scarring.

To prevent smallpox a smoking shovel of hot coals with **sulphur** sprinkled on was carried through the house as an act of fumigation. This method was still being used for cases of **diphtheria** in the early part of the 20th century.

SMOKING. Lighting a cigarette was advised on entering a sickroom and for keeping free of **malaria**. Many could only face using an outdoor privy with a lighted cigarette to combat the smell.

During the First World War soldiers were encouraged to smoke to

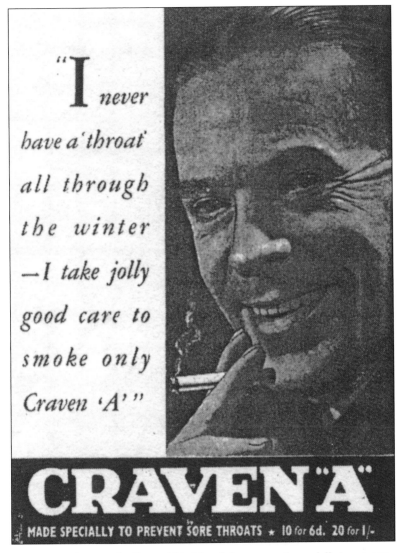

A 1936 advertisement for Craven 'A' claimed, they are made specially to prevent sore throats. Many will have enjoyed smoking thinking they were following a healthy regime, sadly as we now know, it was not so.

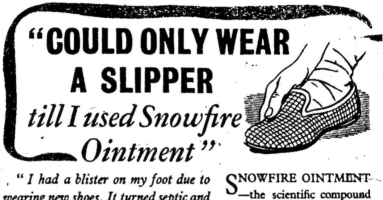

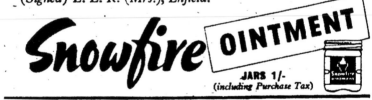

A 1945 advertisement for the popular chilblain treatment Snowfire Ointment.

calm their fear and to help the war effort with extra tax revenue. Advertisements presented smoking as sophisticated and some claimed that their brand of cigarettes prevented **sore throats**.

We are all aware now of the carcinogenic effects of smoking and the advice given in the past seems irresponsible and dangerous. However, there will come a time when some everyday thing we do or eat now will be found to be just as dangerous. Who knows what it might be?

SNEEZE. The words 'Bless you' after a sneeze go back to the time when a sneeze was the first symptom of the **plague**.

SNEEZEWORT. *Achillea ptarmica*. A perennial herb found on damp grassland. Grown here since the 16th century the dried and powdered leaves were used as a kind of snuff. However, it also had medicinal properties that helped with the pain from **toothache** and **rheumatism**.

SNOWDROP. Nature provides this little flower in the darkest days of January and perhaps it is inevitable that it has properties said to be good for illnesses associated with the cold, notably frostbite and **chilblains**. The Lincolnshire bulb industry first started with snowdrops which seemed to grow better there than in Holland. From the 1890s there was a thriving cottage industry, especially round Spalding, Holbeach, Swineshead and Wyberton, of ordinary housholders growing snowdrops for the bulbs which were crushed and made into the popular **Snowfire ointment** for **chilblains**.

SNOWFIRE OINTMENT. A popular patent remedy for **chilblains** and **chapped hands**. See **snowdrop**.

SOAP. Soap was often put into the chemist's handmade pills as a bulking agent. There would have been some antiseptic properties in the soap but the chief result would have been as a **purgative** and in stubborn cases of **constipation** a pellet made of soap was pushed up the 'back passage.'

A soap and sugar **poultice** was good for drawing **boils** or removing glass shards or 'spells' from **cuts**.

See also **blister**, **jaundice** and **opodeldoc**.

SOAPWORT. *Saponaria officinalis*. Also known as 'bouncing Bet.' Who knows the identity of Bet? Perhaps the name is linked in some way to the use of the plant's dried stems and roots in **decoctions** for treating venereal diseases, such as **syphilis** in the past.

Since medieval times the leaves were used for cleaning purposes as soap was not in general use until the 1800s. Country people put soapwort leaves in warm water and agitated the washing with a posser to remove the dirt from the clothes.

The leaves were used in a **poultice** to relieve skin diseases. Soapwort is a powerful herb and would not be advised today as an excess internally can cause paralysis and destroy the red blood cells.

SORES. From a 1930s home remedy book: beat the white of an egg in **vinegar** and sugar and apply to a sore mouth.

Many claimed a drop of warm **mutton suet** or a **poultice** of **watercress** applied to a sore at night would give excellent results.

In Somerset they set great store for healing a sore on applying the cream from the top of the milk, straight from the cow, while it was still warm.

SORE THROAT. This can be a painful part of many illnesses. Mothers used ingredients from the kitchen cupboard and garden, which when sipped were soothing but also astringent, in an effort to reduce the swollen painful tissue. The following were held to be very effective:

A teaspoon of **raspberry** vinegar and **olive oil**.

Elderberry syrup mixed with **honey**.

Garden **thyme** made into a tea.

A teaspoonful of warm **vinegar** sipped very slowly. Other more palatable remedies mixed **vinegar** with sugar or with butter and sugar.

For a good gargle a medicine bottle was half filled with cold **tea** in which you dissolved a teaspoon of salt and a tablespoon of vinegar. A tablespoon of this was then mixed with half a cup of warm water and used as a gargle every 4 hours.

A gargle much preferred by men was whisky, because you could swallow it afterwards.

Any 'theatrical' staying at the Grand Hotel, Scarborough in the 1890s for the summer season who felt a sore throat coming on was always advised by the lady who looked after them to chew a small piece of tangerine peel. See also **tonsillitis** and **blackcurrant**.

Warmth was applied to the throat in a variety of innovative ways. **Goose grease** and red **flannel** or a hot roast potato cut open and wrapped in flannel were left on overnight. Others preferred mashing the potato, wrapping it in a cloth, and placing it in a stocking with a little **olive oil** or **camphorated oil** rubbed onto the outside.

Other sufferers swore by a slice of fatty bacon placed round the neck at bedtime and held in place by the left leg of a stocking; my informant from County Durham did not know why it had to be the left one. By the morning the bacon was cooked and the throat very much better. Some might say an easy way of having breakfast in bed.

Further hot 'fillings' for stockings were blackened burnt **toast** soaked in **vinegar**, warmed and tied round the throat or a hot boiled **onion** cut in half.

A spoonful of **flowers of sulphur** was put into the fold of a clean sheet of notepaper. The one with the sore throat faced a window, opened their mouth and someone else blew the sulphur down the throat. It was always a problem to ensure that the right person blew first!

SORREL. *Rumex acetosa*. Folklore believed that a **decoction** of sorrel leaves would soothe a **fever** and the leaves do have astringent and cooling properties.

SOUTHEND. Southend became fashionable as a holiday resort in 1803 after a visit from Princess Caroline of Brunswick, the wife of the Prince Regent, as she and her daughter Princess Charlotte had been advised to undergo a little **sea bathing** for their health. The local Lord of the Manor Daniel Scratton had every intention of making this a stylish venue and had already built in the 1790s some very fine terraces on top of the cliffs. Alas his plans were scuppered, it was a difficult place to get to and high society failed to visit after the 1830s.

The railway came in 1856 but it was after the Bank Holiday Act of 1870 that floods of Eastenders started arriving. A newspaper of the day referred to them as 'lower classes of excursionists'. The town council of the time insisted the east end of the town, with its amusements and fairs, was specifically for the lower classes and the west end, with its wide promenades, was for the better classes. They preferred to keep them apart.

From the 1870s Southend became known as 'on-Sea' but in fact it is on the Thames Estuary. However, this was an advantage as after the Second World War, London doctors sent their patients suffering from **tuberculosis** or in poor health to walk in the mud as it was thought to be good for them – and it probably was, away from the smog of the city.

SOUTHERNWOOD. *Artemesia abrotanum*. A bitter aromatic herb also known as lad's love or old man. These masculine names may refer to the leaves being supposedly helpful in stimulating hair growth. However, women used the leaves in the form of a tea and it was more widely used up until the 1930s for late or painful menstruation. See also **menses**.

SPANISH LIQUORICE. The dried root of a Mediterranean shrub, *Glycyrrhiza glabra*, used medicinally. Spanish liquorice in hot water was an old remedy for **constipation**.

SPAS. The great age of the spa towns was towards the end of the 18th and the first half of the 19th century when the Napoleonic Wars meant that continental travel was out of the question for those able to afford the luxury of a stay in an elegant European spa town. So instead the unhealthy or hypochondriac rich had to see what England could offer.

Maximilian Hazlemore in *The Family Physician* of 1794 wrote: 'We would advise all who are afflicted with indigestion and want of appetite, to repair to these places of public rendez vous. The very change of air, and cheerful company, will be of service; not to mention the exercise, dissipation, amusements etc. . .'

Many medical men were also entrepreneurs who saw the chance of making money out of the medical tourist. There was no mystery to their cures, although each would claim their own owed much to scientific learning. Pay enough money for a simple diet, fresh air, exercise, plenty of cold water and **purging** and you were bound to feel it was doing good.

Many small market towns with decent water or a saline or chalybeate spring built a pump room and touted for business. Some undoubtedly had quiet charms and fresh air but the key to success was a visit from royalty, without that you were never going to be on the medical map. The purity of the Shropshire water at Church Stretton and the saline springs of Tenbury Wells in Worcestershire were both popular for a short time but failed to rival the spas patronised by royalty and the upper class.

See also **Bath**, **Cheltenham**, **Harrogate**, **Leamington Spa**, **Malvern** and **Tunbridge Wells**.

SPECIFIC. An old word for a drug used to treat a 'specific' disease. See **Royal blood mixture**.

SPIDER. The people of the Somerset Levels suffered greatly in the past from **ague**. An old folklore cure recommended carrying a large spider shut in a box and as it died your ague would lessen. See also **cobweb** and **transference**.

SPITTING. This disgusting habit was constantly seen everywhere and indicated the poor state of the British lungs. Getting rid of phlegm was thought the healthy thing to do at any time or in any place. Public houses had spittoons in which to aim the spit and if you missed, the sawdust on the floor sprinkled there for that very reason helped soak it up.

Spitting was a way of passing on **tuberculosis**, or phthisis as it was called and some attempt was made to control it, especially for those known to have the disease. It was such a problem that it even received royal attention as the Prince of Wales, later to become Edward VII in 1901, formed a committee to stop spitting in places such as railway carriages, theatre and music halls and to prevent 'promiscuous spitting' in all public places.

By the early 1900s, according to the Medical Officer of Health for Erith in Kent, pocket spittoons were issued to all persons suffering from phthisis who required them.

It was still a problem in the 1940s when notices appeared warning of the dangers of spitting in public and advising the use of a handkerchief.

'If you see a neighbour spit
Let the warden know of it.
On this matter please be firm,
Handkerchiefs will stop that germ'.

SPOTS. From a 1930s home remedy book a simple cure: 'For spots and blemishes, apply the juice of **onions** mixed with **vinegar**.' A cloth with **urine** on it was sometimes wiped over a spotty face and this was often done when a baby had a rash.

For spots on the arms and shoulders a Victorian beauty tip recommended rubbing in the juice of a raw greengage. See also **complexion** and **parsley**.

SPRAINS. A **poultice** of **comfrey** leaves or rubbing on comfrey oil was a popular and well known remedy.

John Wesley in *Primitive Physic* recommended cold water or if this failed, 'Mix a little **turpentine** with flour and the yolk of an Egg; and apply it as a plaister [sic]. This cures in a desperate case.'

There were many remedies using basic household ingredients, for example, a cloth soaked in **witch hazel** and wrapped round the sprain, a **poultice** of **bran** and **vinegar** or one made from **mustard**.

In the North and Midlands it was common practice to tie a strand of knitting wool round a sprained wrist or to tie the second and third fingers together.

SPRING TONIC. Thought to be essential for good health after a long dark winter with a lack of fresh vegetables and fruit. The following recipe comes from a very old book, date unknown, produced by the Bavington Presbyterian Church in Northumberland. Put 1 ounce each of **Epsom salts, flowers of sulphur**, cream of tartar and the juice of 3 **lemons** into jug and pour over 1 quart of boiling water. When cold add sugar to taste and take a wineglassfull every morning. This would undoubtedly have acted as an **aperient**. See also **Easter-ledge pudding, nettles** and **watercress**.

If you did not feel like preparing your own tonic, Clarkes Blood Mixture was a very popular springtime patent medicine.

SQUILLS. The bulb of the sea onion found in the Mediterranean that was sliced, dried and used medicinally in **cough medicines** as a powerful expectorant.

STINGS. Bees, **nettles** and ants have acidic stings and are therefore neutralised by the alkaline secretions in a **dock leaf**, especially the smaller 'sour dockings'. However, for increased effectiveness always add some **saliva**. A wasp sting is alkaline and is neutralised by dabbing on **vinegar**. In the past treacle and the juice from the crushed leaves of the **houseleek** were also used. In more recent times mothers moistened the washday 'dolly blue bag', which worked but left odd blue stains on the skin.

STITCH. A sharp pain in the side caused by a muscle contracting and often felt after strenuous exercise. To the highly superstitious people of the Middle Ages the pain was caused by an arrow shot by an elf. The plant **stitchwort** was associated with elves so what was more natural than to turn to the plant for healing.

For the pain John Wesley in *Primitive Physic* advised: 'Apply Treacle spread on hot toast.' By the 1930s this had changed to a mixture of treacle and hot potato. This all seems rather messy and as 'a stitch' goes away on resting it may well be that a continuous pain was something more serious for which the heat gave some comfort.

STITCHWORT. Any number of plants from the genus *Stellaria* and I will not burden you with them all but wood, greater, lesser, marsh, bog, mountain . . . all were thought to relieve a painful **stitch**. Stitchwort was drunk in wine with powdered acorns for the pain and this brew was also said to help if you wanted to have a baby boy. It is unclear whether the mother or father had to drink it.

STOMACH DISORDERS. From the 18th century onwards drinking **sea water** was a universal but doubtful cure. If you could not get to the sea you could always buy a bottle of sea water from Brighton or **Margate**.

John Wesley in *Primitive Physic* unwisely recommended an equally unpleasant glass of **vinegar**.

However, in most houses the more gentle and soothing

chamomile or **sage** tea was enjoyed. An even simpler preparation was half a pint of tap water mixed with the beaten white of an egg. See also **lime**.

STOMACH ULCER. See **ulcer** and **olive oil**.

STRENGTHENING MIXTURES. Chronic ill health, a succession of childhood illnesses, **anaemia**, overwork, major illness, any one of these could leave you feeling listless and miserable. Great trust was placed in the family strengthening mixture for bringing some strength and zest back to the pale and feeble.

Mixtures were recorded in the family cookery book or **commonplace book** and the common link with most of these strengthening mixtures were the large numbers of eggs needed.

Put 6 whole eggs in a basin and squeeze the juice of a **lemon** over them and let them stand for 3 or 4 days, turning over frequently until the shells are dissolved. Then beat together and strain through a sieve into a bottle and add 8 ounces of sugar, quarter of an ounce of isinglass [gelatine], 1 pint of best rum. Shake well and take 1 tablespoon for adults and half for children.

Mix together 6 ounces each of **olive oil**, cod liver oil, 6 well beaten eggs and a large tin of Nestle's condensed milk. Take a dessertspoonful 3 times a day.

A simpler mixture was a raw egg beaten with sugar and milk.

Patent preparations that were popular included Virol, Neave's Food, Easton's Syrup, Fellows' Syrup and Parrishes Food.

STROKE. See **apoplexy**.

STYE. Also called powke, blaine or stine-eye. Sleeping with a rotten **apple** spread over a handkerchief and tied over the eye was said to be a very effective immediate cure or you could substitute cold teabags for the apple. See also **figwort**.

Other methods of soothing and reducing the inflammation were bathing the eye with warm water mixed with boracic powder, a **parsley** poultice or a dab or two of your own **saliva**.

Those seeking a cure in the past were told to rub the stye with a gold wedding ring. In the Black Country they were more precise, it had to be rubbed 9 times to be effective.

SULPHUR. Sulphur has disinfectant and antiparasitic properties and when burned produces sulphurous acid gas. People still recall coming home from school in the 1920s and 1930s and being made to stand over a fire shovel of red hot coals, sprinkled with sulphur. See **diphtheria**.

Sulphur was burnt in the cellar to prevent **malaria**.

From *The Lady's World* 1898: 'When **grippe** or other epidemics are prevailing wear a little crude sulphur in your boots or shoes.'

A spoonful of **flowers of sulphur** was blown down the throat to cure a **sore throat**.

Sulphur was a popular **aperient** taken in the form of brimstone and treacle.

Used externally it cleared up skin diseases like **scabies** and **grocers' itch**. A 1920s home remedy book advised: 'Sulphur baths good for Itch – Travellers and others have much risk to run in having unclean sheets supplied to sleep in. The consequence is some skin disease, such as the itch, tantamount to **ringworm**, for which sulphur baths should be used immediately.'

SUNBURN. A remedy spanning John Wesley's *Primitive Physic* in the 18th century through to the Second World War – wash the burned skin in **sage** tea.

SUPERSTITION. There was a strong belief in magic and charms to cure illnesses right up to the 1920s and in some country areas old ideas hung on even longer. People believed in the magical powers of **transference** so their illness passed to an animal or object and, as well as this, charms, incantations and weird rituals were all considered especially effective in cases of **warts**, **whooping cough** and **toothache**.

SWALLOW OIL. See **celandine**.

SWEET CICELY. *Myrrhis odorata*. Also known as sweet chervil or garden myrrh. It was originally used in cooking as when any part is crushed it produces a strong smell of aniseed. However, it was long regarded as a stimulant for the elderly as it aided digestion and was thought to be helpful in **rheumatism**. The leaves were used in soup and the roots cooked as a vegetable.

SWOLLEN GLANDS. To reduce the swelling **iodine** was painted onto the neck leaving a nasty brown stain. See also **neck**.

SYPHILIS. Commonly referred to for centuries as 'the great pox'. A contagious venereal disease caught by having sexual intercourse with someone already infected. Once it was known as the Neapolitan disease as there was a severe outbreak among the French soldiers beseiging Naples in the late 1400s. In England we called it 'French Pox', reflecting perhaps our deep distrust of all things across the Channel.

Since 1940 syphilis has been treated with penicillin. However, if not treated in time vital organs are damaged and insanity and death follow. This was a disease tackled by the medical profession with salts of mercury and later organic arsenical preparations. Steam baths were recommended. Later the patient was subjected to **malaria** as the resulting fever had some success in halting the disease.

It frequently destroyed lives and the disastrous results were passed on to an innocent wife, who became infected by her husband, and to her children, who were then born with congenital syphilis. Those suffering tertiary syphilis were confined to the horror of a lunatic asylum.

See also **soapwort** and **Royal blood mixture**.

SYRUP OF FIGS. See **aperient**.

T

Keep on good terms with your wife, your stomach and your conscience.

TANSY. *Tanacetum vulgare*, a member of the daisy family. Modern day science recognises that the plant is extremely potent and tansy oil is particularly toxic. Large doses can cause kidney and brain damge. All they knew in the past was the herb had proven abilities to get rid of annoying and debilitating intestinal parasites, in other words **worms**.

Tansy cake was eaten as an Easter reviver after the restrictions of Lent. John **Gerard** in his *Herball* wrote that tansy cakes made with young leaves and eggs: 'be pleasant in taste and good for the stomacke. For if any bad humours cleave there unto, it doth perfectly concot them and scowre them downwards.'

Tansy has a pungent smell which came in useful as a 'strewing herb' and an insect repellant. The leaves were placed under the mattress and between the blankets to kill bed bugs. In Sussex tansy leaves were placed in footwear to keep away the mosquitoes and thereby prevent the **ague**.

A **poultice** of tansy leaves was once used to cure **varicose veins**.

TAPEWORM. A parasitic worm that lives in the human intestine and is caused through eating under-cooked meat or having food or hands contaminated with faeces. In the 1930s the problem was thought to be caused by eating too many potatoes or butcher's meat and milk that had not been scalded.

John Wesley in *Primitive Physic* could not differentiate between the different types of parasitic worm but described the symptoms as: 'A child may be known to have the worms by chillness, paleness, hollow eyes, itching of the nose, starting in sleep and an unusually stinking breath.' He advised drinking any of the following: **salt** water, **nitre** in broth, **lemon** juice, **onion** water, or **quicksilver** in spring water.

From the middle of the 19th century onwards **Whelpton's**

Vegetable Purifying Pills were found to be excellent for these unwelcome guests as one of the ingredients, cambog, a yellow gum resin, was a powerful **purgative** capable of expelling tapeworms. By the 1920s we preferred a few doses of **castor oil** or a worm powder made of **senna** leaves. If that did not work 20 drops of **turpentine** taken before breakfast 'Is a quick destroyer of worms'. See also **benjamin**.

Some society ladies of the 1920s and 1930s were known to deliberately take tapeworms in order to stay thin!

TAR. Tar is a complex substance that has medicinal properties which have an irritating and stimulating effect, acting as an expectorant and making coughing easier. The chemistry was not understood, but people did know that the vapour from tar, especially when it was hot, helped clear chest infections and especially **whooping cough**. Anxious mothers trailed sick children around the town in pursuit of the tar wagon, making them breathe in the fumes at the side of the road.

A lady recalled for me her childhood in Warwickshire in the late 1920s. Here a method of bringing tar into the sickroom was tar yarn tied to the bed head, obtained from the plumber who used it for lagging pipes.

A gentleman whose boyhood was spent in Bradford in the 1930s and 1940s clearly remembered the common use of tar from the gas works. In hot weather the tar melted on the road and you collected it in a tin can from the side of the road. Once home a red hot poker was plunged into the tar and you put a towel over your head and sniffed in the fumes. See also **plaster**.

TAR WATER. Wood tar mixed with cold water. An idea brought back from America in the 1700s and seen as a cure-all, used particularly in the treatment of **erysipelas**, **fever**, **palsy** and **scrofula**. Wood tar contains among other things creosote and carbolic acid which acted as an antiseptic. It was not perhaps the miracle cure claimed by some of its advocates and as it tasted horrid it was a fashion that did not last long.

TEA. 'The cup that cheers but does not inebriate' originally referred to **tar water**. Tea was introduced here in the early 1600s and was thought of as medicinal but was so expensive that it was drunk only by the better off. Samuel Pepys wrote in his diary in June 1667: 'By coach home and there find my wife making of tea, a drink which Mr Pelling the pothecary tells her is good for her cold and defluxions.'

When tea drinking became more affordable for the working classes there was great opposition from doctors and clergymen for a variety of bizarre reasons. It was seen as particularly bad for children under the age of twelve and 'the **female constitution**'.

Country people had always brewed and drunk their own beer – it was safer than **water**. The clergy of the time thought if a housewife no longer spent part of her day making beer for the family she would have spare time for bad habits and loose ways.

John Wesley in 1745 set an example to the poor and gave up tea. 'We agreed it would prevent great expense, as well of health as of time and of money, if the poor people of our society could be persuaded to leave off drinking of tea.'

William Cobbett (1763–1835) the English politician, journalist and champion of the working class, wrote a pamphlet on *The Vice of Tea Drinking*. He predicted that nothing good would come of tea drinking: 'I view the drinking of tea as a destroyer of health, an enfeebler of the frame, an engender of effeminacy and laziness, a debaucher of youth and a maker of misery for old age.'

Even in Victorian times doctors were fulminating against the physical effect of tea, believing it to be 'evil'. Among the many conditions it was supposed to aggravate, a Doctor Browne listed: 'Nervous, bilious, spasmodic and stomach complaints appearing among the lower rank of life.' Even up to the 1920s it was thought to be a cause of short sight!

See also **sore throat**.

TEETH. For centuries false teeth could be supplied – at a price – made from ivory, bone or wood. The latter must have had a limited life and the danger from splinters must have been considerable. Teeth were a nuisance and frequently those setting off for duty in the British Colonies had their teeth extracted before

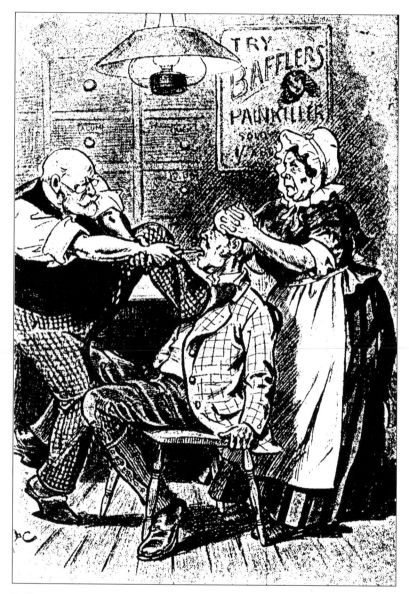

Pulling teeth, or grinders as they were sometimes called required strength and fortitude – and that was just for the one doing the extracting! (Joe Pie Picture Library)

embarking, on the principle that it was one less thing to go wrong. As late as the 1950s I knew of someone who had all her teeth removed as a 21st birthday present.

In the 1920s and 1930s there was a fashionable theory of dental sepsis and doctors believed that bad teeth were the cause of most illnesses. Countless were whipped out and this was a particularly popular treatment of the insane.

When children's milk teeth became loose a popular way, though looking back a bit drastic, of pulling out the wobbly tooth, was to tie a cotton thread round the tooth and attach the other end to an open door. When the door was slammed shut the tooth would pop out.

TEETH CLEANING. Teeth were cleaned with soot from the back of the fireplace or a mixture of **salt** and soot, burnt **toast**, tobacco ash, chewing **lemon** peel or rubbing with a **sage** leaf.

For a homemade tooth powder you mixed chalk powder, attar (an essential oil) of roses, sugar and **bicarbonate of soda**.

To whiten teeth you rubbed them with **honey** mixed with finely powdered charcoal.

TEETHING. Before the Pharmacy Act of 1868 patent medicines containing **opium** could be bought from every corner shop and these medicines were generously used on babies suffering painful inflamed gums. Rubbing the gums with homemade poppy tea was soothing and if all else failed a drop of **gin** in the feeding bottle would knock the child out.

Superstition abounded and even John Wesley felt it had a place in his *Primitive Physic* recommending a necklace of the woody nightshade plant, all parts of which like the deadly one, are poisonous! Other 'helpful' necklaces for round the baby's neck were made from such bizarre items as: moles' claws, acorns, a double hazel nut, coral or anything red.

At the beginning of the 1900s other draconian measures had taken the place of opium. Keeping a baby 'regular' was now the key to trouble-free teething and regular doses of **castor oil** and **Turkey rhubarb** were administered along with a **plaster** made of pitch, a

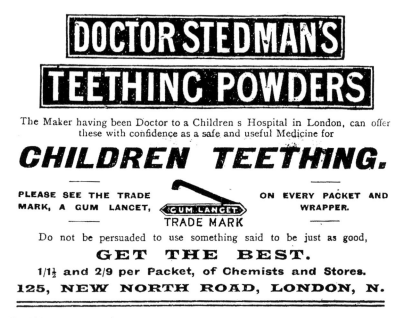

By 1915 people were becoming concerned over the use of narcotics in patent medicines. Dr Stedman's Teething Powders advertisement seeks to reassure.

product of distilling tar, placed between the baby's shoulders and kept there to be renewed once every 2 weeks.

By the 1920s a home remedy book was advocating a more wholesome approach and one which differs little from modern day thinking. 'Teething is a grievous time of trial for most infants. But the child which has not been over-fed, and whose blood has been kept cool by simply taking its natural food, milk, will now receive the rewarding benefit . . . while those babies which have imprudently been stuffed with gravies, pieces of meat, cordial, etc., or have been over-fed, will now greatly suffer, and may, by the indiscretion, perhaps lose their lives.'

THYME. *Thymus vulgaris*. Garden or common thyme has been recognised for centuries as a medicinal plant for its antiseptic and preservative properties, indeed the ancient Egyptians used the oil for embalming. A tea made from thyme was said to be good for **colds** and a **sore throat**. It was also drunk when you were troubled by a recurring **nightmare**.

TINCTURE. Made by soaking fresh or dried herbs in alcohol or a mix of 3 parts alcohol and 1 part water for at least 7 days in a cool dark place, occasionally stirring. The liquid is then strained off and allowed to stand until it is clear. A tincture can be used internally, as a gargle or externally on the skin. See also **inflammation**.

TOAST. Burnt toast is not the useless item you might at first think. Kept warm it could provide comfort for **earache** and was used for **teeth cleaning**.

A Black Country remedy had a cheap cure for **flatulence** using 2 slices of burnt toast. Put the burnt pieces into a bowl and cover with boiling water. Allow to cool and drink. A clever simple way of taking a form of charcoal which is known to cure wind.

TONIC. Most patent medicines contained **paregoric**, a form of **opium** but as people began to realise that these were addictive they preferred the safer alternative and made their own **strengthening mixtures** at home. A **spring tonic** was an essential part of family life and **beetroot** wine was drunk as a **pick-me-up**. See also **Indian brandee**, **quinine** and **under the weather**.

TONSILLITIS. Tonsils are a part of our immune system and protect the body against infection. Up until the late 1930s doctors whipped them out at the drop of a hat. It was such a common and everyday procedure that often the operation, where the tonsils were 'guillotined', took place on the family kitchen table. As can be imagined there were complications and bungling and it was not unknown for children to die after the operation.

See also **sore throat**.

TOOTHACHE. For centuries it was thought that toothache was caused by worms in the jaw. Pulling teeth was a brutal and painful affair (some might say that it still is), so every effort was made to cure the toothache before submitting to a tooth-drawer.

In the 18th century people believed in **transference** of the pain by way of holding a piece of meat to the cheek for 7 hours and then burying the meat. As the meat rotted, so the pain would disappear.

See also **warts**.

John Wesley in *Primitive Physic* provided more cures for toothache than any other illness.

'Lay roasted parings of **turnips,** as hot as may be, behind the ear.'
'A bag filled with hot **chamomile** flowers.'
'Lay bruised or boil'd **nettles** to the cheek.'
'Apply to the face the skin of a Mole.'
'A Sheep's tooth in a bag will cure the pain.'

Maximilian Hazlemore writing in *The Family Physician* in 1794 advised an alarming range of treatments. 'In order to relieve toothache we must first endeavour to draw off the **humours** from the part affected. This may be done by mild **purgatives**, scarifying [see **scarification**] the gums or applying **leeches** to them, and bathing the feet frequently with warm water . . . **vomits** too, have often an exceeding good effect in the toothache. It is seldom safe to draw a tooth till proper evacuations have been previewed.'

There were a large number of toothache cures, reflecting a common problem and a universal fear. Many were in use until the 1960s when our dread of dentists subsided, as their ability to provide painfree dental care and a quieter drill increased.

A numbing effect was achieved by chewing on a **clove** or placing a little grated **horseradish** round the root.

Whisky or **iodine** on cotton wool was rubbed on the tooth and gum or oil of **cloves** or **poppy**.

Warmth lessened the pain and a variety of household items were heated and held to the cheek and ear including:

Warmed **brown paper** sprinkled with **vinegar** and pepper.

A **poultice** of hot **oatmeal**.

A large toasted **cabbage** leaf wrapped in a flannel.

Toothache was a rich seam for the superstitious. From North Yorkshire to Devon there was a general belief that obtaining a tooth from a churchyard and rubbing the cheek with it would charm away toothache.

In Staffordshire they believed that the Devil was responsible and a good living was to be had selling paper charms bearing various incantations to take away the toothache.

In Shropshire they wore a mole's foot round the neck to keep free from toothache.

TORMENTIL. *Potentilla erecta*. Also known as bloodroot. In Latin 'tormentum' means 'torment' or 'anguish'. This is a perennial herb found growing in heaths, bogs and fens. It has powerful astringent and anti-inflammatroy properties and the root is high in tannins and was once used as an **infusion** to treat colitis, peptic **ulcers** and general stomach pains.

TRANSFERENCE. In the superstitious 17th and 18th centuries, and even later in remote country areas, it was widely believed that you could transfer your illness to another person. This seems hardly charitable but was achieved by rubbing a coin on the infected part and leaving it for someone else to pick up.

Toads, moles, rabbits, spiders, snails and dogs were also used for transference, often involving a ritual of some cruelty. However, the West Country idea of a sandwich made from the hair of a child with **whooping cough** and given to a dog seems harmless enough, if not very pleasant for the dog.

TRAVEL SICKNESS. See also **sea sickness**. Travelling great distances was not a pastime open to the poor. However, if you did not want to take a patent medicine, sitting on a wad of brown paper was said to quell the nausea.

Or you could suck a barley sugar sweet.

TUBERCULOSIS. Other names **consumption**, Phthisis or in Victorian England, the White Death or White Plague, on account of the pale skin of those who were ill. Tuberculosis is an ancient disease and found more frequently in medieval England in the form of **scrofula**. However, from the 16th century, as people moved into towns and cities, pulmonary tuberculosis became widespread. By the 1850s 1 in 6 deaths were due to tuberculosis.

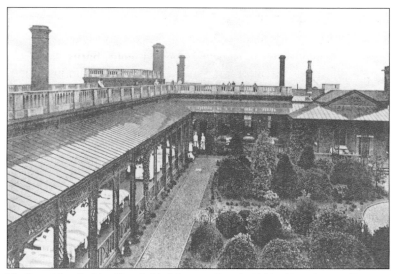

The Royal Sea Bathing Hospital in Margate, Kent in 1905 with patients suffering from tuberculosis in beds on an open verandah for maximum fresh air. (By kind permission of Margate Library, Kent County Council)

Tuberculosis is not just a disease of the lungs but can affect almost any organ. However, the most common form was pulmonary tuberculosis with the dreaded symptoms of coughing, blood-stained sputum, **fever** and the wasting away of the body. The infection is spread by breathing in infected droplets and used to spread quickly in crowded, badly ventilated houses, shops, offices and factories. It was also spread through the milk from cows with infected udders. However, TB was no respecter of persons and the upper class was just as likely to suffer. See **spitting**.

The tuberculous bacillus was discovered in 1882 by the German Robert Koch, but knowing the cause and treating it effectively were two different things. The conditions in which people lived and worked were still as bad and the bacillus thrived. There was no effective cure treatment for consumptives until the 1940s, which brought the discovery of streptomycin and the testing of dairy herds for tuberculosis and the pasteurising of milk.

Dr Benjamin Allen of Braintree in Essex in the 1700s had his tubercular patients steep a pint of sheep's dung in a pint of milk overnight and after straining, drink the liquid as a cure.

John Wesley was acutely aware of the disease and, as so often with his remedies, saw a cure in repeated **cold baths**. He also recommended various remedies with milk as the main ingredient – but we can hardly blame him as milk was seen as a good wholesome food.

His other ideas were odd but at least involved an element of fresh air:

'Every morning cut up a little turf of fresh earth, and, lying down, breathe into the hole for a quarter of an hour – I have known a deep consumption cured thus.'

'Sleep 3 nights in the cow-house, as near to the cow as possible.'

Live snails were eaten in the belief they would consume the phlegm off the chest. The mollusc was everywhere with snail soup, snails in ale and for added 'bite' slugs and earthworms were added. Even as late as 1875 a detailed doctor's cure had as one of the items 2 ounces of mouse ear. They were desperate times.

Cures were sought in **spa** towns and sanatoria. If you were lucky you were sent to a sanatorium outside the town, situated high up where the building caught the winds. There you slept in cold conditions in corridors that were virtually outdoors. The food was frugal and the rooms sparsely furnished. Men and women were kept separately but allowed to eat their meals together. Some sanatoria would only allow a very small amount of boiled milk to be drunk in tea. Others made their patients drink gallons of the stuff – not very helpful if it had not been pasteurised.

Those unable to go away were advised to build an open air shelter in the garden and stay there during daylight hours. This was fine if you had a garden but of no help if you lived in a tenement slum.

Medical folklore had been dealing with tuberculosis for centuries and recommended **rosemary** tea as a restorative, **ginger** to aid the circulation and reduce the fever and coughing, *lobelia inflata* as an emetic and relaxant and **ground ivy** as an expectorant.

See also **aphrodisiac, Margate** and **Southend**.

TUMOUR. See **cancer** and **onion**.

TUNBRIDGE WELLS. This was just wooded Kent countryside until Lord North discovered a chalybeate spring in 1606 and returned to London proclaiming his recovery from **consumption**. Royalty and nobility soon flocked to take the waters which were said to be good for 'Cold, nervous complaints and bad digestion'. See also **menses**.

Building began in the 1630s and throughout the 18th and 19th centuries Tunbridge Wells was a flourishing and fashionable **spa**. That people felt better after visiting Tunbridge Wells was probably more to do with the fresh air and the town's glittering social life, run by its Master of Ceremonies Beau Nash, who arrived from **Bath** to take up residence in 1735.

Like all **spa** towns it was not a cheap place to stay. An extract from the Mildmay Archives shows an Essex gentleman's medical accounts:

1745 August 26. Spent at Tunbridge in 6 weeks, viz., from July 6 to Aug. 16:

	£	s	d
My lodgings at £6 per week	36.	0.	0.
6 coach-horses at £3. 6. 4. per week	19.	18.	0.
9 horses at grass at 18s. per week	5.	8.	0.
Housekeping the 1st week	21.	6.	0.
Housekeeping 2nd week	20.	12.	0.
Housekeeping 3rd week	19.	0.	3.
Housekeeping 4th week	18.	14.	0.
Housekeeping 5th week	16.	17.	6.
Housekeeping 6th week	13.	2.	6.
Gave the dipper for my Lady Fitzwalter and myself.	2.	2.	0.
Gave the maid-servants of the house I hired	3.	3.	0.
Gave to the servants of the 2 great rooms	1.	1.	0.
All expenses included, I spent not less than	£200.	0.	0.

To put this sum in perspective the annual income for at least the poorer half of the population in England at that time was £23 per family. Even lawyers at the top of the earnings scale (nothing changes there!) could only expect a total annual income of £200.

TURKEY RHUBARB. Medicinal rhubarb readily available at the chemist's shop, known as Turkey Rhubarb because it was grown in Turkey. The root of the plant was used as a cure for **constipation** and as a cure-all for everything from an upset stomach to **teething** problems in babies.

TURNIPS. A neglected vegetable now – but not by our grandparents. Sliced it formed the basis of a very pleasant **cough medicine**, hot it gave comfort for **toothache** and applied to the feet reduced the fever of **smallpox**.

TURPENTINE. Oil distilled from certain types of pine trees, known as spirit of turpentine, was a handy home remedy used as an antiseptic for **cuts**, for getting rid of **nits** and as a counter irritant. It formed the basis of homemade **embrocations, liniments** and **plasters** and was rubbed on the chest in cases of **bronchitis**.

Doughty country women sprinkled turpentine onto a piece of blanket and wore it next to the skin inside a corset.

Many elderly ladies favoured a few drops of turpentine on a lump of sugar each day to cure **rheumatism** and for a chest **cough**.

TYPHOID FEVER. Enteric fever is highly infectious and caused by bacteria that live in human faeces, spread by infected food, milk and contaminated **water**. The unpleasant symptoms are a high fever, abdominal pains, dreadful **diarrhoea** in some cases, rose coloured spots and delirium. These symptoms gave rise to the general terms of low fever and spotted fever. Death occurred from either exhaustion, haemorrhaging from the bowels or peritonitis.

The poor in their squalid living conditions were particularly vunerable but no one escaped and it was a greatly feared and little understood illness. Queen Victoria's beloved Albert died of typhoid at Windsor in 1861. This was sad and unfair as previously he had done his best to sort out the unsanitary conditions at

Windsor where in 1844 there were 53 overflowing cesspits under the castle.

Ten years on the Earl of Chesterfield died and the Prince of Wales, later to become Edward VII, almost died of typhoid on a visit to Scarborough staying with the Countess of Londesborough whose defective drains at Londesborough Lodge were the subject of bitter recrimination.

The treatments were those for **fevers**. Typhoid and **typhus** were lumped together and it was only in the middle of the 1800s that Sir William Jenner (1815–1898) discovered the difference.

Typhoid was still stalking the back alleys of cities in the 1920s where primitive collection of human waste from brick-built bucket privies meant infection was easy. It was only with the coming of decent plumbing and sewers that this illness became rarer, a fact that Prince Albert could have told them a century earlier.

TYPHUS. Also known as ship fever and gaol fever, this is an acute infectious disease caused by an organism carried by lice, fleas and ticks. It flourishes in overcrowded, unsanitary conditions and soldiers on campaigns were particularly vunerable. The symptoms were headache, **fever**, a rash, delirium followed by death from heart failure. The treatments were the usual ones for fever and the juice of the **ground ivy** was sometimes given to reduce the effects of the rash.

U

Health and cheerfulness mutually beget each other.

ULCERS. John Wesley in *Primitive Physic* advised 'a poultis of boil'd Parsnips. This will cure even when the bone is foul.'

For ulcers and **piles** a 1920s home remedy book advocated 'the free use of the plant **tormentil** made and used in the manner of tea, sweetened with **honey**.'

From the same book stomach ulcers were treated both internally and externally, 'There need be no better remedy than black treacle and yeast, used in equal parts, and outwardly a little **goose grease**, same time.'

Drinking a glass of **olive oil** while eating was said to soothe a stomach ulcer.

See also **legs, marigold, wood betony** and **placenta**.

UNDER THE WEATHER. An informal expression for not being in the best of health and sometimes used euphemistically for being drunk. It probably goes back to our days as a seafaring country when it meant being on the rougher side of the boat towards the wind.

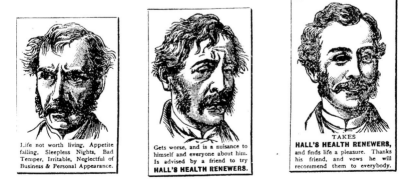

Life not worth living, Appetite failing, Sleepless Nights, Bad Temper, Irritable, Neglectful of Business & Personal Appearance.

Gets worse, and is a nuisance to himself and everyone about him. Is advised by a friend to try **HALL'S HEALTH RENEWERS**.

TAKES
HALL'S HEALTH RENEWERS, and finds life a pleasure. Thanks his friend, and vows he will recommend them to everybody.

That under the weather feeling banished by Hall's Health Renewers which claimed to be 'purely vegetable' – a euphemism for a laxative.

We seem very reticent when describing how we feel, with 'fair to middling' denoting we are neither very well nor very ill, whilst 'very moderate' in North Yorkshire means 'I am practically on my death bed'.

In Tyneside a Geordie would say, 'I'm not ower cliwor,' meaning they were not feeling 'over clever'.

I was told of one mother's no-nonsense cure when anyone was poorly: 'I'll find you something useful to do, it will take your mind off it!'

An old **commonplace book** compiled during the late 1800s advised for the 'under the weather' feeling a porridge made of **rhubarb** and frumenty. Frumenty was a mixture of either pearl barley or **oats** cooked in milk with sugar and nutmeg.

UNDERWEAR. Some children from poor families, even as late as the 1940s, were sewn into their underwear in autumn and not unstitched until the spring. In more respectable houses with middle class pretensions there was an abiding fear of having an accident and on arrival in hospital your underwear being revealed as mucky. People setting off on a journey changed into clean underwear, 'in case I have an accident'.

URINE. From my previous books on the social history of the lavatory I probably know more about the uses of urine than is good for me. It may be a human waste product but in years gone by it was seldom wasted for the chamber pot under the bed held liquid gold. In the garden it went on the soil to feed the tomatoes and **rhubarb** and in the house a splash went into the final rinse when washing blankets – it made them fluffy. In the West Riding of Yorkshire textile mills used urine, known as 'lant' which was collected commercially from willing householders by a carter often with 'Piss' added to his name.

A wash of your own urine was known to clear spots and rashes and West Midland mothers wiped their baby's face with a wet nappy for a bonny complexion.

Coal miners relieved their sweaty sore feet after a hard day down the pit by 'weeing' into a chamber pot and soaking their feet in it until the urine went cold. Urine was good for feet generally, especially for **athlete's foot**, **blisters** and **chilblains**.

During the First World War soldiers urinated into a handkerchief or piece of cloth and held it over their faces to help mitigate the awful effects of the mustard gas.

For urine obstruction and difficulty in passing water a 1920s home remedy book advised drinking lemonade mixed with **dandelion** tea.

See also **cystitis** and **pisse prophet**.

V

Man's best companion – Innocence and Health

VACCINATION. A very negative message was carried in a 1920s home remedy book: 'IMPORTANT – When vaccinating has to take place let it be done at six weeks old; a tea-spoonful of **castor oil** given before and after will carry it safely over. Vaccination has been a means of spreading dangerous and incurable disease.' It is surprising that a popular book used for reference in many households should hold such a suspicious view of vaccination. Yet even today doubts have resurfaced with the continued debate and opposition to the combined MMR vaccination for babies.

See also **smallpox**.

VALERIAN. *Valeriana officinalis*. Also known as garden heliotrope. The name comes from the Latin 'valere' meaning to be well or strong and the plant's sedative and calming properties have been used for centuries for **sleeplessness**. In Warwickshire the root was boiled and used for nervous debility and according to a contempory account, tasted awful. See also **epilepsy**.

VAMPERS. Knitted body belts for children soaked in **camphorated oil** and worn during the winter to guard against childhood illnesses.

VARICOSE VEINS. Said to be caused by crossing the legs, wearing tight garters below the knees and . . . **constipation**. See also **tansy**.

VASELINE. The trade name for petroleum jelly. According to a beautician friend of mine there is a no finer night time face cream than a layer of vaseline. She declined to say how this might affect marital relations. See also **neck**.

VEGETARIANISM. In Victorian times this was seen as an eccentricity reflected in the quote from a President of the College of Physicians, 'Vegetarianism is harmless enough though apt to fill a man with wind and self righteousness.' However, some were beginning to see it as a healthy lifestyle, but generally only by

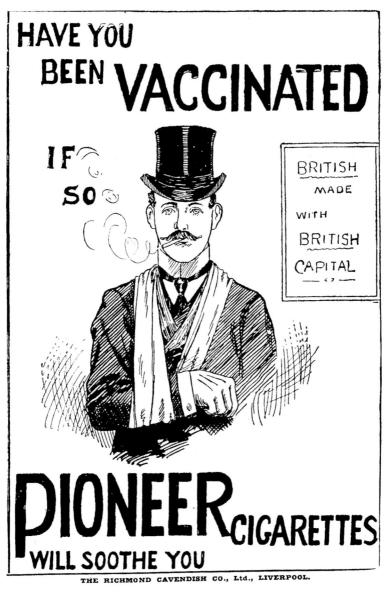

Vaccination was not taken lightly, even needing an arm sling. Again a cigarette was seen as a medical aid for calming and soothing. (Joe Pie Picture Library)

those who could afford to eat meat in the first place. For the poor eating as much meat as possible was their idea of how to keep fit and well.

A 1920s home remedy book wrote glowingly of the benefits of vegetarianism. 'The old monks' and friars' recipe – who enjoyed the best of health, with such cheerful minds – was the use of rice and fruit in preference to animal food of any kind. They lived to great ages, with a fresh complexion to the last.' How could the writer possibly know?

VENEREAL DISEASE. A general term for any infection transmitted during sexual contact. See **syphilis**. For centuries those men who gave it any thought wore a sheath made of sheep gut to protect themselves from infection.

Gonorrhoea, known as 'the clap' was seen by men as an inconvenience which a few hot steam baths would cure. Unfortunately in an infected woman it could lead to sterility. Venereal disease was not discussed centuries ago, any more than it is today.

There was an urban myth, I am sure still around, that unspeakable diseases lurked on a lavatory seat. Mothers instilled such a fear of the undefined nasty diseases lurking on public lavatory seats that even now some of us will go to great lengths never to touch one. There was a story in a national newspaper recently about a Hollywood film star who had thrown a massive tantrum on the film set because someone had used her private lavatory. The newspaper was very critical of this, but with my mother's words ringing in my ears, I had absolute sympathy for the woman!

VERRUCA. The Latin term for **wart**, although we associate verrucas or plantar warts with the feet. The juice of a **dandelion** had the same effect on a verruca as it did on a wart on other parts of the body.

VERTIGO. There were many remedies for 'Vertigo or Swimming in the Head' in John Wesley's *Primitive Physic* but like **dizziness** it could be a symptom of any number of illnesses. John Wesley understood that more often than not it is the result of a problem in the internal ear or a stomach disorder.

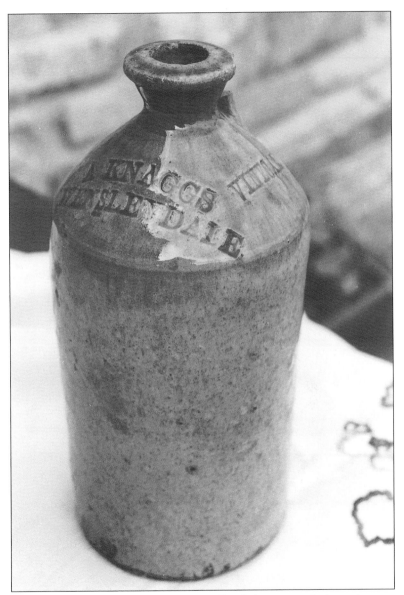

Vinegar was such a popular and useful ingredient in home cures for its astringent and acidic properties that it was bought and stored in large stone jars. (Photograph Ann Holubecki)

'Drop juice of **pimpernel** into ear morning and evening.'

'In a May Morning; about sun-rise, snuff up daily the dew that is on the Mallow Leaves.'

'Apply to the top of the head, shaven, a plaister of Flour of **brimstone**, and White of Eggs.'

'Take every morning half a dram of **mustard** seed.'

'Take a **vomit** or two.'

VINEGAR. During the **Plague** it was used to disinfect money. Tradesmen in towns had a bowl of water and vinegar in which customers would place their money when paying for the goods. In the country, money was left in water and vinegar in **plague stones** on the boundary of a village.

Vinegar has always been valued as a useful household commodity. It was sold in large earthenware flagons and was an ingredient in many home remedies. It was used when nursing anyone with a **fever**, in the treatment of a **cold**, **headache**, **lethargy** or a **sore throat**. See also **alcoholism**.

VISITING THE SICK. Hints for the sickroom from a home almanac dated 1914 advised caution: 'Do not visit the sick when you are fatigued, or when in a state of perspiration, or with the stomach empty – for in such conditions you are liable to take the infection. When the disease is very contagious, place yourself at the side of the patient which is nearest to the window. Do not enter the room the first thing in the morning, before it has been aired; and when you come away, take some food, change your clothing immediately, and expose the latter to the air for some days.' Sound and rigorous advice.

VOMITING. A distressing occurrence which could be due to any number of irritants, indigestible food, **stomach disorders** or dosing oneself too 'heroically' (see **heroic**) on homemade remedies. John Wesley in *Primitive Physic* unwisely advised an **infusion** of **quicksilver** as a way of settling the stomach.

By 1794 a diet of thin gruel was recommended but this sensible advice was followed by the opinion that **oysters**, which at that time were cheap and readily available, should be 'a principal part of the diet'.

For vomiting brought on by 'Violent passions or affections of the mind,' a glass of **negus** or a little brandy and water to which a few drops of **laudanum** might be added.

VOMITS. For any illness the first course of home and professional treatment was always attending to the **bowels** and quantities of **aperients** were given to add to the misery of someone already suffering. If there was no improvement a specially prepared vomit was given to make the patient sick.

John Wesley advised in *Primitive Physic* an **infusion** of either artichoke leaves or radish seed.

An easier but horrid vomit was swallowing **salt** water. However, less drastic and used countrywide was to make the patient drink milk in the belief that it would either make them sick or settle the stomach; either would be a satisfactory outcome.

W

Watercress sellers are the saviours of their country.

WARTS. To any question about warts the answer must be – how long have you got? The cures for warts ranged from the fairly sensible to the weird, and suggestion therapy, wart charmers, poisonous substances, toads, animals and witchcraft were all involved. Warts are certainly disfiguring and no childhood story is complete without a witch or a giant sporting an ugly wart. Judging from the number of cures there were few people in the past who had not at one time or another suffered a wart.

My mother, who came from the Thames Valley, believed that warts were caused by the water in which eggs were hardboiled and

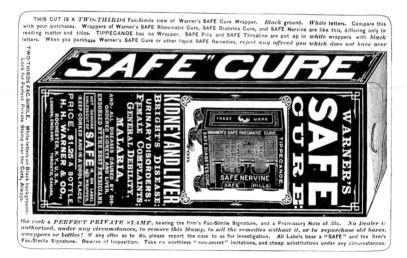

Hulbert Harrington Warner was an American farmboy who after a career selling safes founded his medical company in 1879 at the age of 37. By 1888 he had the largest patent medicine business in the world but four years later lost everything in a Stock Market crash. His cures were far from 'safe' and the ingredients of alcohol, ipecacuanha and extract of mandrake, a highly poisonous plant could lead to death for anyone suffering from Bright's disease of the kidneys. Warner's cures were available up until 1946. (By kind permission of the Thackray Museum, Leeds)

always kept a separate saucepan for eggs. On the other hand a book on Yorkshire witchcraft published in 1773 advised you to get rid of a wart by washing it with water in which eggs had been boiled.

Warts are a virus infection and slightly contagious and are likely to disappear on their own. It is acknowledged that 'suggestion therapy' can be successful in making warts disappear and if the 'suggestion' is cloaked in some odd ritual it will seem all the more potent. The mysterious gypsies were especially good at wart charming but every village and town had its 'wart charmer', who was not necessarily an old woman. The village chemist in Knowle in Warwickshire would charm warts off for sixpence in the 1920s. However, in the West Country the charmer did not want to be thanked as it would undo the charm.

All the remedies collected here have at one time or another worked for someone and whatever we think of them now, anything with an abrasive quality might have been useful.

It was recommended to rub the wart with one of the following: warm **castor oil**, sand, the striking end of a match, the side of a matchbox, the juice from a **dandelion** stem, **euphorbia** (spurge), **houseleek**, or **marigold**. The list is almost endless: a radish, fish liver, mole or swine's blood, **elder** leaves, **fastin' spittle**, the liquid from a horse's hoof boiled in rainwater and finally frog's spit – how would one obtain it?

An unusual cure I have only found in Wiltshire is mother of pearl buttons dissolved in lemon juice and used as a paste.

Other cures required an extra ingredient of 'theatre' and mystique as in the following:

Rub the wart with a cut raw potato and bury the potato in the garden.

Place a piece of raw beef on the wart, wish it to go away, then hide the beef in the garden and do not tell anyone where you have hidden it. As the meat rots the wart will disappear. Yorkshire and Somerset folklore insisted the meat must be stolen first!

However, for the more thrifty, and not to waste good meat, you substituted a broad bean pod for the meat.

Pull out a hair from a horse's tail and tie the hair round the wart and after a while the wart will drop off.

Rub a wart with a black snail then impale the snail on a thorn bush. As the snail dies so too will the wart but you must not let anyone see you do this.

A northern cure involving **transference** advised you to count your warts and into a small bag put an equal number of pebbles. You had to leave the bag where four roads meet and whoever picked up the bag would take on your warts. In Oswestry in Shropshire they substituted grains of wheat.

An interesting cure came from the blacksmith at Preston Park Museum near Yarm, County Durham who has seen it work in very bad cases. A little of the dirty 'bosh' water in which the blacksmith's tools are cooled is taken home in a jam jar and dabbed onto the wart every night.

WATER. A cup of hot water drunk half an hour before a meal was said to prevent **indigestion** and taken regularly would help prevent **constipation**. See also **biliousness**.

However, in the event that this did not work, children with constipation were made to sit on a chamber pot full of hot water, until the water went cold. One assumes that the heat would relax the child but those who remember being made to do this never recalled it being any help.

Unfortunately water was not the pure commodity we like to think our water supply is today, although judging by the amount of bottled water sold, we have our doubts. The coming of piped water into houses or backyards in Victorian times was far from the blessing it seemed at first. The water was taken from rivers into which untreated sewage flowed and was often highly contaminated. Life-threatening illnesses like **cholera**, **dysentery** and **typhoid** together with unidentifiable **fevers** could all be caused by contaminated water.

Upper class Victorian houses had stoneware vessels containing carbon block purifiers to treat their water. The lower classes took to **tea,** as at least the water had been boiled, but many still thought **beer** and **gin** were safer.

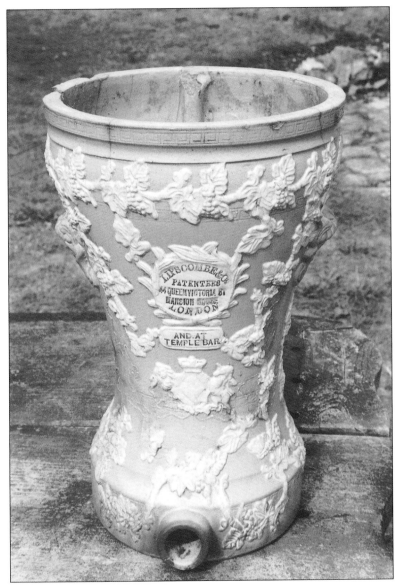

Only to be found in the better class of Victorian household: not a lavatory bowl but a carbon block purifier The water was poured into the top and filtered through, ready to use as drinking water from a tap at the bottom.

WATERCRESS. *Nasturtium officinale* has been known for centuries to do you good. It contains iron, iodine and calcium and is a stimulant plant which clears toxins and is good for almost anything! Without knowing the science, as a 1920s home remedy book quoted: 'Everyone knows the value of the watercress.' It was used as a **spring tonic** and given to those in failing health.

First grown commercially in 1808 at Gravesend in Kent to supply Covent Garden Market it was on sale in all the major cities as an effective ingredient for home treatments. Watercress tea was considered especially good for **whooping cough**. See also **eczema** and **sores**.

WELLS. Holy wells, natural springs and the beliefs that surrounded them are still to be found everywhere, even in this secular age. Springs were known and venerated in pagan times. The Romans first built shrines over their wells and made flower offerings to the gods. Well worship was frowned on by the early Christians but unable to overcome the belief in the water, Christians incorporated the wells as their own. This was followed in the 17th and 18th century by those with an eye for business turning some of them into **spas**. The water often contained helpful minerals and acquired a reputation for healing through superstition, legend or word of mouth. Many wells were early places of prayer connected with a saint or a Christian martyr, whose bones may have rested there on the way for burial elsewhere.

Miraculous cures were claimed for **epilepsy** and the lame but the most common cures were for skin diseases, especially **eczema**, and eye problems. Even recently I came across a 'rag' well in North Yorkshire, still visited for healing, as the fresh handkerchiefs tied to a nearby bush testified. At a 'rag' well a cloth is dipped in the water and then applied to the part needing healing. The 'rag' is then tied to a bush nearby and as it rots you are healed. The cynical might argue that in the time it takes for a piece of cloth to rot you would have got better anyway.

Some wells, often named Bridewell, were thought to increase fertility and newlyweds would drink the water to ensure many healthy children.

The colourful festivals of well dressing still take place in Derbyshire. It is thought the custom of Derbyshire well dressing first started in Tissington in the middle of the 14th century as a thanksgiving for having escaped the **Black Death**.

See also **chalice well**.

WEN. A sebaceous cyst occurring on the face or scalp. In more superstitious times a wen was thought to be cured by the touch of a dead man's hand. See also **public hanging** and **salt**.

WESLEY. The Reverend John Wesley (1703–1791), an Anglican clergyman who together with his brother Charles formed the Methodist movement. His *Primitive Physic* was first published in 1747 and so popular were his remedies that by 1840 the book had reached it 36th edition. 'It is my design to set down cheap, safe and easy medicines, easily to be known, easy to be procured, and easy to be applied by plain unlettered men.' The profits from his hugely successful book went towards the maintenance of Methodist preachers.

His work drew on the medical knowledge of the time but still did not completely eliminate superstition, for how else can we explain his use of a sheep's tooth as a cure for **toothache**. Wesley wrote of his intentions: 'I have once more recommended to men of plain unbiassed reason, such remedies as Air, Water, Whey, Honey, Treacle, Salt, Vinegar and common English Herbs.'

His one aim was to help the poor and at the same time keep them out of the clutches of **quacks**. 'In uncommon or complicated diseases or where life is more immediately in danger, apply to a Physisican [sic] that fears God.' His ideas were used extensively and echoes of his remedies can still be found in the home remedy books of the early 1900s.

WET SHEET. A remarkably uncomfortable **spa** treatment favoured in hydropathic establishments. A patient lay on a bed wrapped tightly in a cold wet sheet and then had blankets piled on top and left for half an hour. This was followed by a cold bath and a brisk rub down. See also **Malvern**.

WHELPTON'S VEGETABLE PURIFYING PILLS. The claim

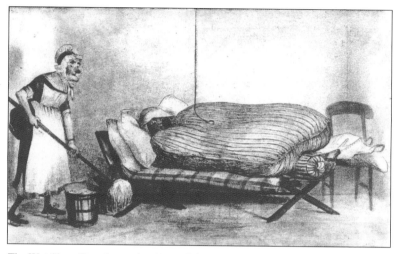

The Wet Sheet Cure from a humorous Victorian booklet *The Sure Water Cure* which referred to this treatment as 'The Mummy State.' (By kind permission of Harrogate Museums and Art Gallery Service)

was that they assisted 'Nature to get rid of superfluous matter', also that a course of treatment 'relieves the congested condition of the skin and kidneys, and tends to restore the natural function of these important organs. For abscesses, boils, ulcers and scorbutic eruptions.' A powerful stomachic containing **aloes** and **ginger**, these pills worked principally as a laxative.

George 'Pills' Whelpton (1797–1873) was born near Horncastle in Lincolnshire and was originally a boot and shoe maker in Louth and a preacher in the Wesleyan Methodist chapel. His wife Elizabeth had continual ill health, perhaps three sons in three years did not help. George studied medical books in the Louth Mechanics Institute and tried various remedies on his poor wife until he found one which led to her recovery. A story has it that he found the famous remedy in the drawer of a piece of furniture bought at an auction. It is thought more likely now that he was given it by another chapel member.

By 1835 the reputation of Whelpton's Vegetable Pills was well established and Whelpton was making the family a fortune. The pills were on sale until well after the end of the Second World War.

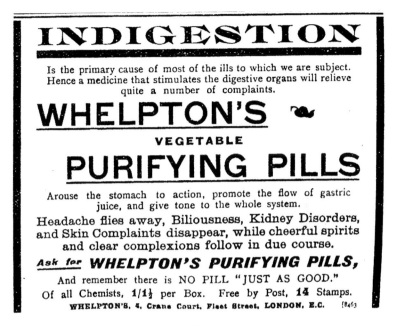

INDIGESTION

Is the primary cause of most of the ills to which we are subject. Hence a medicine that stimulates the digestive organs will relieve quite a number of complaints.

WHELPTON'S

VEGETABLE

PURIFYING PILLS

Arouse the stomach to action, promote the flow of gastric juice, and give tone to the whole system.

Headache flies away, Biliousness, Kidney Disorders, and Skin Complaints disappear, while cheerful spirits and clear complexions follow in due course.

Ask for **WHELPTON'S PURIFYING PILLS,**

And remember there is NO PILL "JUST AS GOOD."

Of all Chemists, 1/1½ per Box. Free by Post, 14 Stamps.

WHELPTON'S, 4, Crane Court, Fleet Street, LONDON, E.C.   [8463]

These 'vegetable purifying pills' helped Whelpton to a fortune and a house in Regent's Park, London. Later he instigated the building of St Saviour's church in Eastbourne, where his son became vicar, and also funded The Whelpton Almshouses in Horncastle, Lincolnshire.

WHITES. *Fluor Albus* or nowadays known as leucorrhoea, a vaginal discharge. One might be surprised to find that John Wesley in *Primitive Physic* tackled this subject full on and did not flinch from what was a very private condition. It is caused by infection anywhere in the genital tract and was a debilitating illness suffered by many women.

Wesley advised sleeping on your back, eating moderately and the inevitable purge. After the purge followed a recommendation to take either **quicksilver** or **antimony**; both were highly dangerous. Antimony is poisonous if taken in large doses and would have produced violent vomiting, more purging and even death. I cannot help thinking the misery and violence of this remedy might somehow be seen as a punishment.

Thankfully 50 years on *On the Diseases of Female* published in

1841 advised gentler measures – drinking **sarsaparilla** mixed with dill water.

WHITLOW. A pus filled inflammation of the finger or toe and sometimes referred to as a **gathering**.

John Wesley in *Primitive Physic* thought a cure lay in binding the whitlow with either a horse hair, the leaf from a leek or a piece of 'rusty Bacon'.

As time went on mothers preferred the painful treatment of a hot bread **poultice** applied to the site of infection.

WHOOPING COUGH. Also formerly known as hooping cough, chin cough or kink cough. The hacking cough develops into a distinctive 'whoop' noise as the breath is drawn in at the end of a spasm. It was a distressing illness, often with vomiting after the coughing and a very real danger of **pneumonia**. Whooping cough was once part of every childhood and because it was so common it shared with **warts** more superstition and odd cures than any other illness I have written about.

John Wesley in *Primitive Physic* advised rubbing the child's feet with hog's lard and **garlic** or rum and keeping them warm in front of the fire together with a spoonful of brown sugar and the juice from **pennyroyal**. If only he had stopped there, because his other advice fully subscribed to the 'odd ritual' theory:

'Fill a little muslin bag full of spiders, tie it round the neck of the patient, who wears it night and day, and the cough will disappear.'

'Swallow 4 wood lice alive, in a spoonful of jam or treacle, and the 'whoop' will vanish.'

There was little to chose between these and the whooping cough cures to be found in the Bedale witchcraft book of 1773, which claimed a cure when a skinned fieldmouse was made into a small pie and eaten and the warm skin bound hair-side against the throat and kept there for 9 days.

Certainly people treated whooping cough as they would have done a cough. A 19th century cure for whooping cough from Wiltshire mixed a newlaid egg in half a pint of **vinegar**, followed 36 hours later by 8 ounces of **honey** and a dessertspoonful given to the child when necessary. However these pleasant remedies were not enough, there was something about this illness that demanded more.

A **donkey** featured regularly in the old cures. Taking a child away from the rest of the family was a good idea to stop the spread of the infection and a ride on a seaside donkey would have done no harm but the donkey mystique seemed to be more part of the cure than the sea air. In many counties a child was passed under the belly of a donkey, although in Cumbria and Shropshire an ass or a piebald pony would do just as well. A slight variation had the child riding the donkey across a bridge facing backwards towards the tail!

Symbolism was in every cure. In the Black Country a child was passed through a hole in a growing tree or had a raw potato hung round the neck and as the potato shrivelled the child would recover.

In Staffordshire the Lords Prayer was written out and placed in a little bag round the child's neck. If that did not work the child was made to look at a new moon and say:

> 'What I see may it increase,
> What I feel may it decrease,
> In the name of the Father, Son and Holy Ghost.'

An example of **transference** had the child spit on a piece of meat and the meat was then given to the dog to eat, thereby transferring the whooping cough to the dog.

Or you could catch a frog, open its mouth then cough into it 3 times and then throw the frog over your left shoulder.

Pipefish, also known as needlefish, caught by the fishermen of the River Medway in Kent, were much in demand as a cure. The dried pipefish was grated and a small amount given to the child with jam or honey, which made the child sick and provided relief from the 'whoop'.

People who lived in remote country areas were highly superstitious and none more so than those living on the North

Yorkshire Moors and the east coast. There was a widespread belief in Hobs, a kind of small hairy goblin, right up to the 1900s. A child suffering from whooping cough was taken to the cave called Hob Hole in Runswick Bay, just north of Whitby and at the entrance the mother asked for help:

> 'Hob Hole, Hob,
> Ma bairn's gotten t'kink-cough,
> Tak it off, tak it off!'

A similar ritual took place on the sands between Redcar and Saltburn in Cleveland when the mother carried the child out to the water's edge at low tide and recited: 'Bairn's got kink cough, Tak't off, tak't off,' and walked back slowly with the incoming tide. In both these cases the fresh air must have done some good.

At Ludlow Castle in Shropshire and Haddon Hall in Derbyshire children were taken to ask: 'Echo, please take away my cough.' It is hard to know now to whom they were appealing.

There was plenty of bracing air on any moorland and a child was taken there to be cured of the 'whoop'. A hole was cut into the turf and the child's mouth held close to the freshly dug earth to breathe in the smell which was said to effect a cure. An added refinement in the West Country was that a sheep had to have been lying there.

Fresh air was free and every industrial town had a high point or hill within walking distance where a child was taken to 'blow' away the whooping cough. With the coming of the railways a train journey with the window open, especially in a tunnel, would do just as well.

There was no end to the inventive uses of the industrial processes with which townspeople were surrounded. Miners' wives had the child taken down the pit. Others carried the child through the smoke of a **lime** kiln, some preferred breathing the smell from the gas works and the **tar** on the road was always a favourite. An alternative for those living in the Black Country was to take the child through a canal tunnel. Some children in the North East were put on barges that dumped the nightsoil from Middlesbrough out to sea. The sea air and the methane gas were seen as a winning combination.

Country children got off lightly as their cure was to sleep in the cow byre with the cows, as the strong smell of ammonia from the urine helped their breathing.

By the 1920s most of these odd cures had lapsed in favour of a dose of **castor oil** and syrup of **rhubarb**, for even if you could not cure the 'whoop' you were not going to add **constipation** to the child's troubles. Immunisation against whooping cough began in the mid 1950s, although it was not so long ago that an elderly Cumbrian recalled that he had cured two children by giving them warm milk from a mare.

See also **watercress** and **hawkweed**.

WILD STRAWBERRY. *Fragaria vesca*. I have memories of picking wild strawberries on the disused railway line of my childhood village in Cumbria. The fruit, leaves and roots have digestive and tonic properties and were all used for medicinal purposes.

An **infusion** of the leaves was a treatment for **gout**.

Rubbing the leaves on the face was said to give a young girl a beautiful **complexion**.

WIND. See **flatulence**. A possibly apocryphal tombstone warning known to every schoolboy and used as an excuse when breaking wind in company:

> 'Where e'er you be
> Let your wind be free,
> For holding it back
> Was the death of me.'

One of the most popular patent remedies at the beginning of the 1900s was Page Woodcock's Wind Pills. It is unclear whether the pills were for trapped wind or for creating wind for the ingredients were a powerful combination of **aloes**, **chamomile**, **ginger**, **ipecacuanha**, **peppermint**, **rhubarb** and powdered Castile **soap**.

WINDS. Commonsense advice for the elderly from a 1920s home remedy book. 'Winds (North East) have a very trying effect on all ages, especially those advanced in years; when these winds prevail, simply make free use of **toast** and water, drunk very hot, sweetened well with brown candy, which acts on the lungs.'

In 16th and 17th century Sussex they thought the opposite for they believed the south wind brought sickness and the north east wind brought health.

WITCH HAZEL. *Hamamelis virginiana* or Virginian witch hazel. As the name suggests the Pilgrim Fathers, on settling in Virginia, discovered the Native Americans using the liquid from the bark soaked in water for bruises.

Distilled witch hazel was a staple item in every medicine cupboard for its astringent properties and was used for **sprains**.

See also **mint**.

WOMB. This organ and 'the peculiar function of re-production which it is destined to perform,' was seen by medical men in the past as the root cause of women's illnesses. It was this that made us constantly 'Prone to derangement of health'.

John Wesley in *Primitive Physic* referred to a prolapse of the womb as a 'Falling' and his cure was the same as for **fundament**.

WOOD BETONY. *Stachys officinalis*. Also known as hedge nettle. A perennial herb found in woods, hedges and by the sides of streams. It was once very important in herbal medicines for **wounds** and a 1930s home remedy book felt it was a 'Herb worth knowing . . . one physician found it to cure no less than 47 different diseases.' Unfortunately the book did not go on to list them.

The stems and leaves are astringent and drunk as an **infusion** acted as a tonic. In small doses it had a calming effect in **cystitis** and **diarrhoea** but too much could lead to **vomiting**. It was much prized in Northamptonshire, where 'wood bitney' or 'water bitty', as it was called, was used for external healing and mixed with fat made into an ointment for **piles** and **ulcers**.

WORMS. See **tapeworm** and **gin**.

WORMWOOD. *Artemisia absinthium*. This is an old herb with many medicinal properties but unfortunately it is habit forming and can cause brain damage. The name wormwood comes from the Anglo-Saxon word wermod from which the word Vermouth is derived. Oil of wormwood was once used to flavour both vermouth and absinthe, the highly alcoholic, addictive and – if enough of it was drunk – hallucinatory drink, first made by Henri Pernod in 1797. The use of wormwood in alcoholic drinks was banned from the early 1900s. In a less intoxicating form an **infusion** was once drunk to cure **melancholy**.

WORT. An old name for any plant that was once used medicinally.

WOUNDS. Our forebears had detailed knowledge of the healing properties of plants first discovered by the Ancient Egyptians, the Greeks and the Romans. The early Church used plants and, for those sceptical about their healing properties, some did work. The leaves were bound onto a wound and those mentioned most often for healing were: **agrimony**, **comfrey**, **golden rod**, **ground ivy, herb robert**, **marigold**, **pennywort**, **wood betony** and **yarrow**.

The fishermen and dredgerman of the River Medway in Kent, known as Bawleymen, believed the oil from rendering down the livers of stingrays was very good for treating **wounds** or **burns**.

In many counties they believed that healing would only come if the instrument that had caused the wound was either cleaned thoroughly or rubbed with fatty bacon and the expression used was 'salve the weapon not the wound'. See also **yarrow**.

WOUNDWORT. See **yarrow**.

X Y Z

Excess calls in the doctor

YARROW. *Achillea millefolium*. Also known as woundwort and carpenter's weed on account of the plant's abilities as a **decoction** to heal **wounds** from sharp instruments. It has been known for centuries as a cure-all because of its antiseptic and anti-inflammatory properties.

Yarrow tea was said to be good for **colds** and **rheumatism**.

A sniff of its leaves was said to stop a **nosebleed**.

YEAST. This is a ferment high in vitamin B obtained from brewing beer and when every household brewed their own there was plenty left for the bread making. It was used in the treatment of **colds** and **boils**.

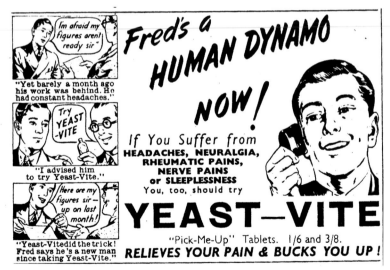

A 1949 advertisement for a much needed tonic. The Second World War may have ended but postwar Britain was a dreary place beset by shortages and still undergoing rationing.

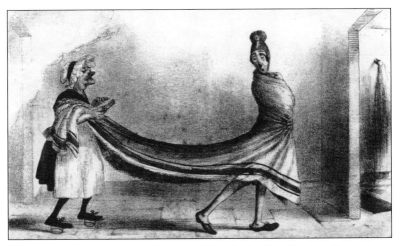

Procession to the Bath. From a humorous Victorian booklet *The Sure Water Cure*.
'Between Steam and Water the Patient protects her feet with straw shoes and hair
in an Oil Skin Cap. A train bearer holding her Blanket, she goes to the cold Plunge
bath where she remains till she warms the water and catches cold.'
(By kind permission of Harrogate Museums and Art Gallery Service)

YELLOW DOCK. *Rumex crispus*. Also known as curled dock.
Once used extensively and especially recommended by
Culpepper, the plant, found on cultivated as well as waste ground
has astringent and tonic properties. A 1920s home remedy book
recommended an **infusion** of the leaves if you could not get any
rhubarb as it would have the same effect but at the same time it
would also clear the skin.

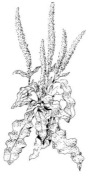

Yellow Dock

ZAM-BUK. A favourite patent medicine at one time used as a healing skin ointment. People made their own from **eucalyptus oil, swallow oil** and **vaseline**.

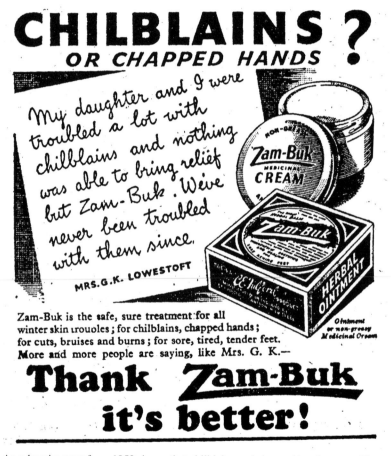

CHILBLAINS ?
OR CHAPPED HANDS ?

My daughter and I were troubled a lot with chilblains and nothing was able to bring relief but Zam-Buk. We've never been troubled with them since.

MRS. G.K. LOWESTOFT

Zam-Buk is the safe, sure treatment for all winter skin troubles ; for chilblains, chapped hands ; for cuts, bruises and burns ; for sore, tired, tender feet. More and more people are saying, like Mrs. G. K.—

Thank Zam-Buk
it's better!

An advertisement from 1952 shows that chilblains and chapped hands were still a problem. Zam-buk was universally admired but many people preferred to make their own from a mixture of eucalyptus oil, swallow oil and vaseline.

Bibliography

PRIMARY SOURCES

The Reverend John Wesley's treatise on medicine, *Primitive Physic*, first published in 1747.

The Family Physician – Being a collection of the most valuable and approved Prescriptions by Mead, Sydenham, Tissot, Fothergill, Elliot, Buchan, and Others by Maximilian Hazlemore, London, 1794.

On the Diseases of Females by Thomas J. Graham MD, 1841.

Family Medical Adviser by John Skelton, Senior. Physician, Surgeon &c, 1866.

The commonplace book of Mr Edward B. Brown of Bainbridge, North Yorkshire 1895, kindly supplied by his granddaughter, R. Cloughton.

Practical Medical and Commercial Recipes by J.T. Butterworth, Qualified Dispenser to the Society of Apothecaries 1897.

The Lady's World, 1898–1899.

600 Valuable Home Recipes – Foundation of Good Health and Happiness – Save Doctors' Fees, published Middlesbrough early 1920s and kindly supplied by M. Nolan.

A Book for Every Home by S. Walker, published Ilkeston, Derbyshire, 1923 and kindly supplied by C. Chippindale.

Every Housewife's Guide Book, compiled by A. Worthington, published Blackpool early 1930s and kindly supplied by B. Marsh.

OTHER SOURCES AND BOOKS OF INTEREST

The Royal Horticultural Society Encyclopedia of Herbs and their Uses, Deni Bown 1995.

Curious Cures of Old Yorkshire, Dulcie Lewis, 2001.

Life and Tradition in the Lake District, William Rollinson.

Pills and Potions – Folk Medicine in the Black Country, John Brimble.

The Bawleymen, Derek Coombe, 1979.

The Book of Gillingham, Norman Tomlinson, 1979.

Hidden Essex, Stanley Jarvis, 1989.

Superstition and Folklore, Michael Williams, 1982.

The Folklore of Cornwall, Tony Deane and Tony Shaw, 1975.

The Folklore of Somerset, Kingsley Palmer, 1976.

The Folklore of Wiltshire, Ralph Whitlock.

Bygone Northamptonshire, William Andrews.

Book of Old Cures and Remedies, Kate Wills and The Living Memory Group, Northampton.

Shropshire Folk-lore, edited by Charlotte S. Burne, first published 1883, reprinted 1973.

A Dictionary of Sussex Folk Medicine, Andrew Allen.

The Blackcountryman Magazine, editor Stan Hill.

English History from Essex Sources 1500–1750, A.C. Edwards, Essex Record Office publication no.17.